Topic of Cancer

Topic of Cancer

Fiona Castle

with
Jan Greenough

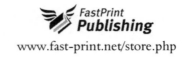

www.fast-print.net/store.php

Topic of Cancer
Copyright © Fiona Castle and Jan Greenough 2012

MICHAEL COZENS
20 ROEDICH DRIVE
TAVERHAM
NORWICH
NR8CRB

ISBN 978-178035-255-8

First published 2012 by
FASTPRINT PUBLISHING
Peterborough, England.

Contents

Foreword

Many years ago I was a regular exhibitor at The Christian Resources Exhibition in Surrey, which always ended with a party arranged by the organisers. One year we were entertained by Roy Castle and his band, who had just launched a new album at Ronnie Scott's in London. At that time Roy was very ill and needed regular rest periods. I had the enormous pleasure of speaking to this remarkable man (and his loving wife Fiona) between numbers. Despite his cancer he impressed me with his cheerfulness, banter and obvious joy in life and in what he was doing. The memory of that meeting has remained with me ever since.

When I was diagnosed with inoperable and incurable prostate cancer in 2004 I decided I would face it like Roy. After three years of treatment I took early retirement but I wanted to keep busy, so I offered my services to help organise a Relay for Life event at Ascot racecourse to raise funds for Cancer Research UK. That action introduced me to a whole new career, working with cancer charities to raise awareness and funds for continued research and support. I have never been so busy or rewarded both emotionally and directly. I found that there was a great need for people with a cancer experience to review publications, give talks and media interviews, campaign, fundraise and bring new ideas to the table.

In 2010 and 2011 I received a series of appointments: as a Cancer Research UK 'Ambassador'; a Macmillan Cancer Support 'Cancer Champion'; and for the American Cancer Society 'International Hero of Hope' and 'Global Cancer Ambassador'. This recognition is humbling when I look at the people I work with and for, but my message to others with this illness is that cancer is not the end – it can be the beginning of a new, wonderful, fascinating and rewarding life.

I could see that locally there was a sad lack of support for patients and their families and carers. Relay for Life enables people affected by cancer to meet to chat with professionals, experts and others who understand their situation. Inspired by this, I decided to start a group meeting monthly to provide these facilities. I called it 'Topic of Cancer' and I am flattered and delighted that Fiona should want to use that name as the title of her book. I wish her every success with this book and her continued work in memory of an equally remarkable man, Roy Castle.

Nigel Lewis-Baker

Author's note

I should like to thank the many people who have helped me in the writing of this book, especially all the patients who talked or wrote to us, some of whom I have mentioned in these pages, who so willingly shared their experiences of cancer.

Most of all I'd like to thank Jan Greenough for her tireless research and her writing skills: this book is born out of our friendship, shared faith, long collaboration and our experiences of cancer among our own families and loved ones.

This book was first published in 2000 by Hodder and Stoughton Ltd, with the title *Cancer's a Word, Not a Sentence*. After a few years it went out of print, and the title was subsequently used by Dr Robert Buckman for his book published by HarperCollins in 2007. Meanwhile, I was constantly being asked at cancer support groups and charities where people could obtain a copy of our original book, so we decided to update it and reprint it – and to avoid confusion we gave it the new title *Topic of Cancer*.

All the profits from the sale of this book will go to the Roy Castle Fund for Cancer Research UK.

Fiona Castle

Introduction

The idea for this book came about because of my concern for the way many people are told their diagnosis: 'I'm sorry, you have cancer.' I visit lots of patient support groups and hospitals, and so often I see people sitting white-faced in waiting rooms, stunned with shock and fear. Too often such patients do not have a support system of specialist cancer nurses to help them pick up the pieces, and provide the wide-ranging information they need. I long to comfort them: to sit down beside them and take their hand, to tell them that I know what they are going through, and that there is hope.

Ideally there should be specialist nurses at every cancer hospital in the country. For every form of cancer it is important that friendly, experienced help should be available to guide people through their diagnosis and treatment.

This book is designed to offer some of that help. It aims to provide basic information in layman's terms, to explain how to absorb the news and to deal with people's responses to it. Because my husband Roy suffered from lung cancer, I have had my own experiences of this disease. I know what hard work the various treatments can be, but how worthwhile when they restore someone to health. We saw the emotional effects on the whole family of learning that Roy was ill, and we found our own ways of coping with it. Those ways may not be the same as yours, but sometimes it helps just to know that others have walked along a similar difficult road.

There are many forms of cancer, so it is not possible to cover each in detail, but at the back of the book you will find a list of the names and websites of useful organisations. Many of them have free telephone helplines.

This book is designed primarily for patients and their families to read and refer to. If it can help, in the initial stages of a diagnosis, to prepare anyone for what may lie ahead, then it will have succeeded in its task.

Part I

Standing Still

Cancer is so limited ...
It cannot cripple love.
It cannot shatter hope.
It cannot erode faith.
It cannot destroy peace.
It cannot kill friendship.
It cannot suppress memories.
It cannot silence courage.
It cannot invade the soul.
It cannot conquer the spirit.
It cannot steal life.

1.Taking It In

Each year in the UK there are a more than a quarter of a million diagnoses of cancer. This book is written for those people, who have been told that they have cancer. Every one of them will have his or her own story, of how the symptoms which were troubling them finally persuaded them to go to the doctor, the various tests, the growing suspicions which they tried to push away, and the eventual realisation that the diagnosis had to be believed: they had cancer.

Many people report that at that moment the world seemed to stand still. Julie Walters, the actress, said of the moment her daughter Maisie was diagnosed with leukaemia, 'The world just stopped.' Cancer is probably (along with AIDS) one of the diseases most feared in the modern world. Yet as my husband Roy used to say, 'Cancer's just a word – not a sentence.' It is a fact that more than one in three people will develop some form of cancer in their lifetime, but it is no longer the death sentence it used to be. Thanks to continuous research, getting better all the time. Many people, after being diagnosed with cancer, may still enjoy ten, twenty, thirty or many more years of active and enjoyable life.

Nevertheless, cancer is a disease which in the popular imagination remains a killer – so much so that when my husband Roy was diagnosed, he found that many people would not even say the word, but referred to it as 'the big C', 'that illness', or even, irritatingly, as 'your little problem'.

Because of this, being told you have cancer is a shock. That moment when the world stands still is a moment when you stand still, too, and feel possibly more alone than you have ever felt. Roy said that after he was told about his lung cancer, 'That five miles' drive home was the loneliest I have ever experienced.' When he, in turn, told me, I felt numb from shock. My thoughts went round and round in circles, as I tried to grasp all the implications at once. Was he going to die? Could the treatment help him? How would we tell the children?

Doctors and nurses

At least Roy was called to the hospital to be told the news in person, by a kindly and sympathetic specialist. I have since spoken to many people who heard about their condition in less considerate ways. Elvira Lowe, who had breast cancer, was telephoned late at night by her consultant, who did not ask whether she was alone at home with no one to talk to. One man, who had no idea what was wrong with him, was sitting in a crowded hospital waiting area when his name was called: 'Mr. Smith, please go over there to the lung cancer specialist.' Some people have been admitted to hospital for tests, and are told about their diagnosis during a routine ward round – they, at least, have nurses with them on the ward who can answer some of their questions and provide some reassurance. Others may be told the news abruptly by a doctor who either uses evasive words ('You have a small growth ...') or hides behind a string of such confusing medical terminology that he might as well be speaking Greek.

Doctors have, presumably, entered the medical profession because they want to help people: they are not intentionally cruel or unfeeling. Yet over and over again I hear stories such as these, when patients are given shattering news in a hurried or off-hand manner which prevents them from asking questions or even being able to think clearly about what is happening. Many doctors feel that medical students still do not receive enough training in communication skills. The doctor who shows by his words, manner, or touch, that he or she has sympathy for you as an individual, can make the news easier to bear.

At this moment of crisis, you don't want to feel that you are being treated as an object of medical interest. You are not just a body with an interesting collection of symptoms, but a real person, with a personality, a life and relationships that are being touched by this news. Anyone who understands and respects your feelings at this moment can be of real help and support.

16

Very often that kind of personal support is more easily found from the nurses. When you are given distressing, alarming information about what is happening to your body, you need intelligent, informed, sympathetic support, and nurses are ideally placed to give that. Many people find them more approachable than doctors, and feel less awkward about asking questions and taking up their time. (The doctor, after all, probably has a whole string of timed appointments which he has to fit into his clinic.) And nurses often have more day-to-day experience of getting alongside patients and talking to them in language they understand.

It is obviously distressing if patients are given devastating and frightening news in a blunt, embarrassed fashion by a busy doctor who is preoccupied by the long clinic he has to get through. Patients should not have to walk out of a consulting room through a waiting room full of other people, and then go and stand at a bus stop while they are still reeling and confused. Best practice suggests that people should be able to leave the doctor and go to a separate, quiet room with a nurse, where they can cry, ask all the questions they need, have a cup of tea, and leave only when they feel ready. They should be able to take with them the telephone number of a nurse who specialises in their form of cancer, who will be willing to answer queries and provide understanding, support and information at any time.

Asking questions

Even if you had already been fearing the worst, once those fears are confirmed you are likely to feel a mixture of shock and disbelief. Many people report a dream-like state: 'I couldn't believe it was really happening to me,' or 'I kept thinking that in a minute I'd wake up.' The knowledge that you have a serious illness which may be fatal completely reorganises your view of the world. For both the patient and the family and friends, our idea of the future is suddenly changed: we are all forced to think about our own mortality – something we tend to avoid most of the time.

It is the quality of this shock which makes the doctor's task more difficult. Many people, when they are told they have cancer, find it impossible to take in anything else. At that point they cannot make decisions about possible courses of treatment, or assess how they might feel about possible side effects.

Because of this, many doctors keep information to a minimum at this session: they know that the patient will probably not remember much. People vary in the amount of information they want: some trust the doctor's skill and have very few questions. Others prefer to ask questions and gather as much information as possible. Yet others want to shut out the news and hide from it, and do not want to have the details explained to them; a doctor who is aware of this may tell them very little.

All of these reactions are normal, but there is often a great deal that you need to know. There are choices and decisions to be made, possibly including your consent to further investigations and treatment. However, your treatment may not start immediately, and there will be time to absorb the news, think about it and come back with questions. We were lucky in having a GP who was also a friend. He visited us at home and answered all our questions frankly. Roy always asked for 'the absolute truth with no cushions'.

Even if you can't think of any questions immediately, you will almost certainly think of many later – usually in the middle of the night! The answer is to jot them all down as they occur to you, and take the list with you the next time you see your doctor. If you still feel that you are too upset to take things in properly, get a friend or family member to go with you, take a notebook, and make notes of what the doctor says. You may feel rushed when you are talking to the doctors, or feel guilty at taking up too much of their time. But it is important that you understand what is happening, and you have a right to the information you need.

Some questions you may want to ask include:

- What kind of cancer do I have? What stage is it at? Has it spread anywhere else?

- What tests do I need? What are they designed to find out? What do they involve?

- What treatment is available for this kind of cancer? What choices do I have?

- Where will I have to go for treatment?

- How will the treatment affect me? What risks and side-effects are there? Will I still be able to work/look after my family?
- How long will the treatment last? How often will I have to have it?
- Will I die?

First reactions

People react in various ways to the news that they have cancer. Roy's first response was to ask questions, to make sure he understood exactly what his situation was. When he got home and told me, a friend was waiting for him to record a 'voice-over' for a fund-raising video: he had to go straight into another room with his script and get down to work. This was typical of him, and throughout his illness he was always keen to do as much work as possible – partly so as not to let people down, but partly because it took his mind off his illness and enabled him to go on doing what he usually did.

While Roy was recording, I stood in the kitchen and leaned against the radiator to try to get warm; I felt chilled and numb. My thoughts went round in circles, and I prayed the sort of desperate, helpless prayers that come in such circumstances. 'Why is this happening? What's the meaning of all this? Lord, how are we going to get through this?' I didn't feel angry with God: I don't believe that illness is sent from God or that he does things to punish us – disease is just a fact of life in the world we live in. After a while I began to feel calmer, and as though God was surrounding me with his love.

When the recording was over, and Roy's friend had gone home, we just held on to one another and cried. For the next twenty-four hours or so, every time I looked at Roy I burst into tears. I simply couldn't take in the news that my strong, healthy husband had a life-threatening disease. The other instinct we both shared was to pray. As Christians, we believed that God cares deeply for us and for everything that affects us. We knew that He was grieving with us for the pain we were going through. Somehow that gave us strength to face the future, and a feeling that we were not alone.

When we told Benjamin (our youngest child, then aged eighteen) he looked, as Roy said, 'seriously transparent', and then we all cried again. Antonia, on the other hand, got angry. Her defiance also seemed to strengthen Roy's resolve to put up with the treatment and get well.

Some people say that they are actually relieved when they are given a diagnosis. They may have been feeling ill for some time, and trying to shake off their fears as well as their symptoms. Sometimes they feel better for knowing that they have a real illness that can be treated, and that they are not just imagining it!

A typical example is Victoria Kagi, who was diagnosed with bone cancer. She started to write poems to express her feelings.

> Then the longest week of my life
> Waiting for the result.
> A phone call:
> It's cancer.
> He said a long name.
> He said 'You have a chance.'
> Our lives stopped somehow,
> They turned upside down.
> I cried,
> I was confused,
> Angry,
> Distraught.
> My three children!
> How, what, when –
> I couldn't think.
> Then people started to pray.
> I told my friends – they prayed.
> I don't know if I prayed,
> But God was there somehow, holding us in his arms.

I wholeheartedly agree that the longest week is the one spent waiting for the results of tests. The day Roy's results were due I couldn't swallow even a cup of tea. Once I knew the results, even though it was not the news we wanted to hear, I felt I could begin to come to terms with it and deal with what was happening to us.

Some people's sensation of disbelief extends into a refusal to think about their illness at all. This is sometimes called 'denial', and the suggestion is made that the ostrich 'hiding your head in the sand until it goes away' approach is somehow harmful. It's true that the cancer is not just going to go away, but there is no need to force yourself to face up to everything all at once. Denial is a normal and healthy method of dealing with overwhelming news, and it seems to serve as a sort of buffer to protect us from collapse. If the news is too big to deal with, we try to shut it out – only of course we can't shut it out entirely, so what really happens is that bit by bit we begin to get used to the idea. Deep down we are moving slowly along the path towards accepting the truth, without being completely overcome by it. Denial becomes a problem only if it goes on for too long and begins to cut us off from communicating with our family and friends and doctors. A few days or weeks of not wanting to think about it will do no harm. As with so many things, you have to work to your own timescales.

Once they have accepted their diagnosis, many people may begin to blame themselves – especially if there is a known cause for their cancer, such as the connection between smoking and lung cancer, or between sunbathing and skin cancer. This is sad, because even though such links have been made, they may not necessarily be the cause in your case: Roy suffered lung cancer and he had never smoked, though he worked in a smoky atmosphere. And anyway, guilt is not a helpful emotion: you have enough to cope with, without adding blame to your burdens.

Anger is another common response. Sometimes people are angry with their doctors for not finding their cancer sooner; some feel angry because the treatment is making them feel ill; others simply become so stressed by the diagnosis that they become irritable with family and friends and take their anger out on them. This is understandable, but of course it can make others wary of getting into conversation with you. It may help to be honest about your feelings, saying, 'I'm sorry if I've been short-tempered, but I keep worrying about this.'

On the other hand, anger is a perfectly reasonable response, and it may give you extra energy and determination to beat your illness.

Telling others

In the past many cancer patients would not be told their diagnosis directly; doctors would talk vaguely about 'a lump' or 'a growth', and sometimes did not even write the word in the patient's notes, in case someone saw it. Occasionally doctors would tell the family the diagnosis but not the patient. This is no longer the case. Nowadays patients expect to be told the truth about their condition, and there is much more information available for them. They have the right to know what is wrong with them: whether they wish to tell their family and friends (or have their doctors and nurses tell them) is up to them.

Lynn Faulds Wood, the television presenter, told me,

When I was diagnosed with bowel cancer it was a bolt out of the blue. I had never heard of the disease, yet it is the second biggest cancer killer after lung cancer. Being told I had cancer was a terrible shock. Even worse was telling my husband, John Stapleton, telling people I loved and seeing the effect on them.

In many ways, it is worse for family and friends than for the person who is going through the disease. We have a job to do, tests and operations, cancer to fight. Our family and friends feel powerless to help, feel guilty perhaps that it hasn't happened to them, and they can suffer terribly without good support.

Some patients are so afraid of the effect the news will have on their family that they try to protect them by keeping it to themselves. This is fair enough where friends and acquaintances are concerned (though you may be passing up a good source of help, support and friendship), but it is seldom a good idea with husbands, wives and the rest of the immediate family. They may be shocked and upset, and afraid to talk about the subject for fear of upsetting you, but it is nearly always better to share the news together.

It is important to be honest, especially between partners. If the facts are not shared, the way is open for misunderstandings, regrets and guilt. In any case, in close relationships it is almost always impossible to keep a secret as big as this. Those who have tried are invariably found out: the biggest give-away is that arguing stops! One man knew only that his wife had been having some tests, but he guessed that she had cancer when she stopped nagging him about mowing the lawn – in the face of serious illness, the minor irritations of everyday life, that used to seem so important, simply shrink away. It is part of the different perspective on life which cancer often brings, and which many cancer patients speak of with some surprise.

When facing cancer, both the patient and the carers need support, and they can often support each other a great deal simply by talking and sharing their fears and worries. People with no one to confide in are much more likely to suffer from depression, which adds another weight to the burden of illness.

On the other hand, we all know that our families are not natural angels of mercy, who can be expected to take on a new role as towers of strength to support us overnight! They will respond to the news in many ways just as the patient has done: with fear, disbelief, anger, or depression. They may be afraid or unwilling to talk about it, possibly just at the time when the patient needs most to talk to someone. They may also feel guilty – perhaps because some of their fears are as much for themselves (how will they cope with your illness?) as for you. Or perhaps they feel what is know as 'survivor guilt' – why did this happen to you and not to them? How can they get on cheerfully with their everyday life when you are in hospital having treatment?

All these mixed feeling can lead to irritability and arguments, just at a time when no one is equipped to deal with them or discuss things rationally! Certainly there were times during Roy's treatment when he would be bad-tempered (which was quite uncharacteristic). In the end we agreed with the family that we all had to give one another space for whatever emotions we had, and that we would try not to over-react or blame each other.

Talking to children

The desire to protect others from the fears and uncertainties of cancer is especially strong where children are concerned. We all want our children to be happy and free from care and worry, and we don't want to have to introduce them to the realities of illness if we can help it. However, we often need to tell them what is happening, and we have to decide what to say according to their age and level of understanding. Children differ in their ability to understand things, so it's important to give them a chance to talk, so that you can check how much they have understood.

It is important to remember that anxiety is always worse than knowledge: children are very sensitive and may be worrying more than you think. Your absence in hospital, your tiredness or illness, or even a series of doctor's appointments, may have already roused their suspicions that something is wrong. Being told the truth, that you are ill and that the doctors are trying to make you better, will enable them to face their fears with your support.

One thing to be especially careful of is children's tendency to think that everything that happens in the world revolves around them. They may think that things have gone wrong because of something they have done or failed to do. It may help to repeat that your illness is not their fault. Small children invariably need the same information to be repeated several times, which can be trying if you have had to wind yourself up to talk about it at all. You need to be very patient while they are absorbing the facts, perhaps over several days or weeks.

Older children may be better able to understand the facts of cancer, but adolescents are often struggling with their own emotional development and their need to grow away from you and become independent. Your illness may add an extra confusion to their feelings: they want to develop their own social life or spend time on their own, but they feel guilty for not wanting to stay by your side. They may be happier talking to other adults outside the family whom they trust, rather than trying to discuss their feelings with you. Their anxiety may be expressed in difficult behaviour, either at home or at school, and this will also require patience and understanding.

Both you, your family, your friends and your carers need time to take it all in. Give yourselves plenty of time to come to terms with what is happening, and don't expect anyone to cope with everything all at once. Eventually you will have to make decisions about treatment and look to the future, but it may be enough for now just to accept that you have a serious illness. But what kind of illness is it, how does it develop, and how can you improve your chances of recovery? Almost certainly, what you want next are some facts.

2. Facing the Facts

What is cancer?

We talk about cancer as though it were a single disease, but in fact there are over 200 different types of cancer. However, the basic problem is the same in all of them. Normal body tissue is made of small building-blocks called cells, and throughout our lives these cells grow and divide to make new healthy tissue. Cells usually divide in a controlled way, but sometimes they change, and go on and on growing and dividing until they form a lump of abnormal tissue: this is called a tumour.

Cells divide by splitting in two, so one cell becomes two, two cells become four, and so on. Each time the cells divide, the number of cells doubles. The speed at which cancer cells divide varies according to the type of cancer, but on average the size of a tumour can double in about a month. This why, once cancer has been diagnosed, it appears to grow quickly. A single cell is microscopic, so if two or four or eight cancerous cells multiply, the whole tumour is still tiny. A clump of one million cells is about the size of a pinhead: no one could see it in the body with the naked eye. On average, cancer is about two and a half years old before it becomes detectable.

Some tumours are harmless (sometimes called 'benign'): they don't spread to other parts of the body, and if they have to be removed by surgery (perhaps because they are pressing on another organ, or because they are unsightly), they usually don't grow again.

The dangerous (or 'malignant') tumours keep growing, and can invade nearby organs and stop them working properly. Also, cells from these tumours can break away and travel to other parts of the body.

Sometimes they travel through the lymph vessels. Lymph is a colourless, watery fluid which bathes all our body tissues and

26

contains a kind of white blood cell which helps the body to fight diseases. The lymph nodes or glands are situated all over our bodies, and they are joined by lymph vessels which eventually drain into the bloodstream. The cancer cells can travel through these, and also through the veins and arteries of the bloodstream, to other parts of the body. There they may start another site where abnormal cells start growing. This is called a metastasis or secondary growth. The original tumour is called a primary growth.

Cancers are classified according to the site where they originated: the most common are carcinomas, which originate in the lining cells in body organs and skin. Sarcomas originate in the structural tissues (muscles, tendon, bones and cartilage); lymphomas come from the lymphatic system and leukaemia from the white cells in the bone marrow.

The causes

Why the cells suddenly start dividing in this uncontrolled way is not properly understood yet. A great deal of research is going on into this, because if we understood the causes of cancer, we might have a useful tool for preventing it. Some general causes have been recognised, but it is generally thought that the development of cancer is very complex. People can be exposed to cancer-causing substances (called carcinogens) for long periods, but their bodies' natural defences may be able to destroy them before any damage is caused to their cells.

Some known carcinogens occur naturally in the world around us: exposure to the ultra-violet wavelengths in sunlight can cause skin cancer. We cannot avoid sunlight entirely, but it is generally accepted that lying on a beach in the hottest part of the day, without wearing sunscreen cream, and especially if we are fair skinned, is unwise. Nowadays in the UK summer weather forecasts often include warnings about the strength of the sun.

Another natural hazard is radioactive material. People who work with radioactive substances are subject to strict regulations and have to wear badges which detect the amount of their exposure.

Man-made substances such as pesticides and other chemicals are also carcinogenic: farmers and others are encouraged to take great care when handling them. Perhaps the most common carcinogen is tobacco, yet many people voluntarily choose to smoke, in spite of all the information now available about its dangers.

Some chemical food additives are thought to be carcinogenic; charred and smoked foods contain nitrites which can be changed into carcinogens in the body; and certain foods such as alcohol and diets rich in fats and salt, although not carcinogenic in themselves, are thought to create the conditions which encourage the growth of cancer cells.

A very few, rare cancers are thought to be caused by viruses, and some by hormonal upsets.

It is clear that we are all exposed to some of these factors at different times in our lives, and yet not everyone develops cancer. It may be that most of the time our immune system is able to control the development of abnormal cells. Why it sometimes fails to do this is yet another unknown. It is possible that the gradual decline in effectiveness of our immune system with age is responsible for the increased likelihood of cancer in older age groups.

Some people believe that extreme stress can cause the body's natural defences to let us down – but again, many people suffer stress without this result. In particular, there is a tendency to recall some stressful event (such as divorce, bereavement or even a burglary) which occurred shortly before the cancer diagnosis. However, as we have seen, cancer has usually been developing for a long time before it is diagnosed – usually since long before the event which is being blamed.

Symptoms

Because there are so many different forms of cancer, which can affect almost any part of the body, the range of symptoms is wide. In addition, the central parts of most organs of the body have no nerve endings, so it is quite possible that no pain is felt until a tumour has grown so large that the outer lining of the organ is stretched. However, there are certain symptoms which always require investigation, even if they may be caused by something quite different and minor. It is always better to err on the side of caution – even if you have already been diagnosed with cancer, it is worth being aware of these signs:

- unusual tiredness and weakness
- sudden weight loss
- fever
- nausea
- sores or scabs which refuse to heal
- lump or change in breast shape
- bleeding or discharge from nipple
- vaginal bleeding between periods or after the menopause
- hoarseness
- difficulty in swallowing
- coughing up phlegm with blood in it
- frequent severe headaches
- blood in urine
- change in shape or size of testes
- change in bowel habits
- abdominal pain.

Reducing risk

Nothing can guarantee to prevent cancer, but there is some standard advice for reducing the risk. It is never too late to follow these guidelines: your cancer may be cured, and you will want to reduce the risk of it recurring. Obviously, reducing the risk is closely connected with avoiding those substances mentioned above which are thought to play a large part in the development of cancers.

Perhaps the most effective step anyone can take to avoid cancer is to avoid smoking: cigarette smoking is known to be the cause of nearly all lung cancers, and the risk increases with the number of cigarettes smoked. However, if a person stops smoking the risk decreases again: after fifteen years, the ex-smoker's chances of developing the disease are very much reduced. Lung cancer is probably the most preventable of all the cancers. Smoking is also implicated in cancers of the bladder, pancreas, larynx, mouth, oesophagus, pharynx and kidney.

Another obvious step is to avoid occupational hazards such as contact with certain chemicals and pesticides, asbestos, nickel, chromium and uranium.

Maintaining a healthy weight and keeping active can help avoid a range of general health problems associated with being overweight, as well as reducing the risk of certain cancers such as breast, kidney and colon.

Limiting your alcohol intake is also wise: heavy drinking (especially in association with smoking) increases the risk of cancers of the mouth, larynx, throat, oesophagus and liver.

Guidelines for diet have also been developed. These are designed for healthy living generally, not just for reducing the risk of cancer, and they cover three main areas:

- avoiding those foods which contain significant levels of carcinogens (such as charred, smoked and cured foods), and highly processed foods containing many additives and colourings
- avoiding those foods which are thought to provide an environment which encourages the growth and spread of cancer cells (such as red meat, alcohol, fat and salt)
- choosing to eat foods which contain nutrients and other compounds which seem to enhance the body's natural defences (such as vegetables and fruits, wholegrains and pulses).

You are bound to want to do everything you can to try to prevent your cancer from recurring, and I have outlined some of the ways in which you may be able to reduce your risk. But what about the disease you currently have? Everyone's biggest question is, 'How can I improve my chances? How can I improve the odds on my recovery?'

Taking the tests

Your first active step is to co-operate with the doctors. You will probably have had a number of tests before you were told that you had cancer. When the diagnosis has been made, it seems strange that often the first thing the doctor does is suggest that you have yet more tests. However, these are extremely important, as they may tell the doctors a great deal about your type of cancer, how advanced it is, and what kind of treatment will work best.

The number of tests you have, how long they take, and how often you will have to go to hospital, all depend on what sort of cancer you have. They may include blood tests, X-rays or scans. The various scans available include CT scans (cross-section images which are analysed by computer), MRI scans, (which produce a picture using radio waves), ultrasound scans (which use sound waves to build up a picture of the organs), mammograms (X-ray pictures of breast tissue) and isotope scans (which use injection of a weak radioactive substance to allow viewing with a special camera). A biopsy involves removing a piece of tissue for examination. An endoscopy involves looking inside the body through a small fibre-optic tube.

None of these is painful, and only the biopsy may involve an anaesthetic, though you will be offered a sedative for an endoscopy. (A general anaesthetic makes the patient deeply unconscious, so that they cannot feel pain; a local anaesthetic numbs a specific area of the body. A sedative makes you feel very relaxed and sleepy, but still conscious.) Roy could remember nothing of his endoscopy afterwards, but the doctors assured him that he had been laughing and joking throughout. He said he wished someone had written it all down, as there might have been some new material for his cabaret act there! On the other hand, the test he hated most was the CT scan: it involved lying quite still in a large tube-like machine, and although completely painless, it made him feel claustrophobic. The man who had fearlessly abseiled down cliffs, taken a 'death slide' from the Blackpool Tower, and wing-walked across the English Channel, was afraid of lying still for five minutes in a hospital scanner. He was offered a sedative for this test, too.

Waiting for the results of tests, like waiting for an initial diagnosis, can be stressful and worrying. However, all these tests can enable the doctors to work in a more focused way, and design the most effective treatment for you.

Getting the best care

If you are not happy with what you have been told, you are entitled to ask for a second opinion from another doctor. In fact it is rare for there to be any major differences of opinion between cancer specialists – those differences which do exist are often in areas where research has still not provided us with sure answers. They are unlikely to make a crucial difference to the outcome of your treatment. But there are some cases where general surgeons have thought a case incurable, but a specialist, who is more familiar with the latest developments in cancer therapies, has been able to recommend a successful treatment.

In some British cancer centres, the treatment is as good as anywhere in the world, but sadly the provision is patchy. Most cancer advice services tell patients that they should always ask whether the doctor they are referred to is a specialist in their type of cancer. Research indicates that specialist care can improve the effectiveness of treatment dramatically, but traditionally, patients in Britain are diagnosed and treated in general hospitals by general doctors and surgeons, who may see only a few cases of their type each year.

The good news is that this picture is changing rapidly. In 1995 the Chief Medical Officers for England and Wales, Sir Kenneth Calman and Dr Deirdre Hine, recommended that British cancer care should be reorganised. Dedicated cancer units for the more common cancers are being set up in district hospitals, and specialist cancer centres providing high-standard, specialised care for most cancers (including rare ones) are being set up in regional centres. Meanwhile, taking an active interest in your own treatment (or getting a confident friend or relation to ask the awkward questions!) could significantly improve your chances.

If you feel able, and if you are the kind of person who wants to know what is going on, contact one of the many cancer charities and support groups listed at the back of this book for more help and advice. When you go to the hospital, ask how many cases of your kind of cancer your surgeon operates on each year – is it enough to make him an expert? How many cases does your doctor deal with, when he is planning the particular cocktail of drugs that are right for you? How expert is your radiotherapist at planning the right doses for this cancer in this part of the body? Is there a case for asking to be referred to another consultant at a different hospital? You may have to travel further, but there is a chance that you might do better there.

The power of positive thinking

Another practical step you can take to improve your chances is to take control of your feelings. At first they were probably running wild, with panic and fear uppermost! After that you may have felt low and depressed, or as though the hospital and the doctors were taking over your life. When you are suffering from a frightening and serious illness there is probably very little that is more irritating than to be told to 'think positively'. People who suffer from depression get equally tired of being told to 'pull themselves together'. If it were possible to snap out of depression simply by making a proper effort, that illness would disappear. Similarly, if it were possible to conquer cancer by the power of thought alone, the hospital waiting room would be a lot emptier. We should always be suspicious of anything that claims to be a certain cure, and this is no different.

Nevertheless, the links between our minds and our bodies are not fully understood. Some doctors claim that particularly determined patients have succeeded in achieving aims they would have thought impossible (such as dancing at a daughter's wedding or climbing a mountain!) and can put this down to nothing other than strength of will. So there may be something in the advice to take a positive attitude. If nothing else, it may make you feel a bit better!

We all know how a worrying pain bothers us. If we suspect that it might be something serious, we are constantly aware of it, trying to measure its intensity, or perhaps planning how we will describe it to the doctor. Once the doctor has listened to us, and has said, 'That's just indigestion from the medication you're taking', it's amazing how the pain recedes from our consciousness. It may still be there, but because we are no longer afraid of it, it no longer seems important, and we are better able to ignore it. Positive thinking changes our perception of the problem, so effectively it gets smaller.

There is more to it than this, however. We know that cancer cells are killed off not only by medication, but also by our immune systems, and we know that our immune system reacts to stress and both mental and physical trauma. It seems likely that we use a certain amount of energy coping with our fears and worries. If we are too distressed, we will have less energy left to fight off diseases – and that includes minor viruses as well as cancer. So how do we come to terms with cancer and stop being afraid of it?

In a sense we can't: it is a serious illness and we are right to be concerned by it. Trying to hide from the facts doesn't help. But we can get it into proportion. No one knows what the future holds for them. We may suddenly feel cheated because our future seems to have shrunk, but in fact no one can be certain of living for another ten or twenty years – we just all live as though we could. We may feel cheated because we are no longer able to run for a bus, or even do our shopping unaided, yet thousands of disabled people live their lives with those restrictions every day.

The fact is that we all live our lives one day at a time, and today is the only reality for everyone. All our planning and arranging for the future doesn't change that. So while we have today, we can live in it, whatever it holds, whether we feel well or ill.

When Roy's cancer was first diagnosed he was about to make a series of programmes for television in America. He was disappointed that this had to be cancelled because his treatment had to start at once – but he jumped at the chance to make a programme in a BBC series called 'Fighting Back'. The programme focused on his illness, but he saw it as a chance to continue working, and also as an opportunity to be open about the disease and clear away some of the fears and misconceptions people had about it. It helped him to retain a positive attitude if he felt he was doing something constructive.

Of course there are times when simply carrying on and ignoring it isn't possible. There are times in the thick of the battle with difficult treatment when it demands your whole attention. And there are times when you just feel low, and can't help feeling sad about the fact that you have cancer. But you can try to make sure that you don't dwell on those feelings for too long. You can choose to think positively – not because you should, or you have to, or because anyone else tells you to, but because you have decided for yourself that is how you will deal with it. Having even this amount of control may help you to regain a feeling of control over the whole situation. You are no longer helpless in the face of illness: you are making your own decisions.

Your mental attitude may not affect the eventual outcome of the illness, but it will almost certainly affect your experience of having the disease. During the 1970s and 1980s Dr David Spiegel ran a support group for breast cancer patients. They were never told that attending this group would affect their survival: it was simply something designed to help them cope better. He duly reported on the results of the experiment, which suggested that those women who attended the support group felt that they had a good quality of life – more so than those who didn't attend. This report (published in 1981 in the Archives of General Psychiatry) found that for this reason it was worth offering support groups to such patients. However, some years later the doctor followed up the same group, and found to his surprise that the survival rate of this group of women was noticeably higher than those who had not attended (this was published in 1991 in the Lancet). Possible reasons for this may be that having the support of the rest of the group encourages women to learn more about their illness, so that they get good treatment and persevere with it; or that their stress and anxiety are significantly reduced. There is now more research going on in this field: at the moment I know of no other research to support these findings.

Roy always used to say 'Don't ever give up! Cancer hates positive people!' Many people all over the world told him that his positive attitude had encouraged them in their own fight against cancer, and he became for many cancer patients a symbol of their determination to beat the disease. Although Roy died of lung cancer, I don't feel that it ever won: right to the end he retained his joy in living, and his thankfulness to God.

If you have a faith, one practical thing you can do is to pray. Many people reading this book may not be Christians, or indeed hold any faith at all, yet many of them will confess that at the hardest times, they have prayed – perhaps a wild, wordless prayer to whoever might be out there. As our wonderful friend Harry Secombe used to say when he was fighting in the Second World War, 'You don't find many atheists in the trenches!'

I am sure God knows and understands these feelings, and the desperation which makes us call out and reach out for any help and support. He never turns His back on any of His children who call out to Him, but is waiting like the father of the Prodigal Son in the Bible, searching the horizon for the first glimpse of our willingness to come home to Him.

Prayer and meditation can have real measurable effects in the clinical sense: a racing pulse can slow, blood pressure can be reduced, and settled calm and tranquillity can bring sleep to the wakeful. Yet these are not the reasons why we pray! Often we pray because we can't help it – even if we don't have the words, or if we are beyond sorting out theological arguments about who Jesus Christ was or is. We just turn to someone who knew what it was to suffer, and who said 'I will never fail you nor forsake you.'

Sometimes that security can be as good as medicine.

3. Support Systems

Modern life has many advantages, but there is no doubt that nowadays we are often more cut off from our neighbours than we would have been a hundred years ago. When we hurry to work or to the shops by car, there is less opportunity to stop and chat in the street; when we spend the evening in front of the television or computer we are less likely to engage in conversation even with our own family, let alone with friends. Add to this the modern emphasis on individual self-sufficiency, and it is little wonder that it does not come naturally to most of us to ask other people for help. Some of us are so much more accustomed to helping others – whether it is through the local charity shop or some other voluntary work – that we seldom stop and ask ourselves what help we might need. Or we may be busy, successful or ambitious at work, with no time to be aware of any needs of our own. Being ill can change our outlook in many ways, but we may still find it difficult to realise that at a time like this we need the support of other people.

Even if you have succeeded in asking questions and getting some basic information about your illness, you may still find yourself hesitating to talk freely to your friends or colleagues about it. Some people report that they felt 'dirty' or 'ashamed' when they heard they had cancer. This is a strange reaction, since cancer is not infectious (you might as well be afraid of catching someone's broken leg!) and it certainly is no one's fault, yet these feelings are very common. Many people told Roy that they were glad that he had made his cancer public knowledge, because until then they had felt embarrassed about talking about it. Other people are so overwhelmed with fear about the illness that they can hardly bear to think about it, let alone talk. Often they have a kind of superstitious feeling that once their fears are spoken, they may come true.

These feelings may have no logical foundation, but they are very real, and they go some way towards explaining why so many people find it difficult to talk about cancer. Yet talking can be very important: we need information and all kinds of support: physical, emotional, spiritual, practical and financial. It may go against the grain to ask for help, but if we want to have the best possible chance of recovery, we need to access all the help available to us.

This does not mean that you will instantly become enfeebled, relying on others to do everything for you. Rather it is a very sensible step to look around and see what kinds of help are available, and what you might require as your needs change. At first you may want someone who can give you reliable information about what is happening ; later you may need someone to accompany you to treatment sessions and perhaps drive you home. Later still you may find that the greatest help comes from others who have had the same illness and similar treatments, who can share your experiences, tell you what it feels like, or even pass on tips for getting over difficulties. So what are the main sources of support available to you?

Using your doctor

The doctor is bound to be your first line of support, mainly as a source of information. We have already said that the appointment for diagnosis is a bad time to try to tell the patient much, but the later appointments for treatment offer more opportunities. Hospitals have changed a great deal in recent years. The old-style National Health Service of the 'Carry On' films, in which the doctors were like gods, and the Matron was if anything even more important and terrifying, has gone. As Claire Rayner once said to a doctor in a radio interview, 'Our parents and grandparents were the people you did things to. We are the people you do things with.' (Radio 4, Today Programme.) Nowadays we expect to be partners in our treatment.

Take along your list of questions, and don't be afraid to ask anything – no question is silly if you want to know the answer. However, it is still true that doctors may have a limited amount of time available, and some confess that their hearts sink when a patient pulls out a long list of questions. Be selective: when you have questions about your own case and your personal situation and symptoms, ask your doctor. When you want more general information, look around for informative leaflets and library books, or turn to the internet – but be wary about the sources you use. Trust the recognised cancer charities or websites used by doctors (like patient.co.uk) and steer clear of sales gimmicks. Nurses can often point you to other sources of information as well as answering your questions themselves. Some nurses will sit in on consultations with you, and then come outside afterwards and check that you have properly understood what you have been told.

We all know how easy it is when talking to our doctors to come away feeling dissatisfied. Sometimes we try to avoid complaining, so we make our symptoms sound milder than they really are – and then we worry that the doctor may not have realised that we really are concerned about that nagging pain. Or alternatively, the doctor may appear to dismiss our symptoms as unimportant, failing to explain to us that they occur regularly in this situation, and will certainly go away soon. Given the level of anxiety on the part of the patient, and the fact that the doctor cannot possibly provide us with detailed accounts of everything that is going on without enrolling us for a degree in medicine, it's not surprising that the exchange of information doesn't always work out.

The main thing is to be as factual as possible. Resist the temptation to sound either brave and stoical ('It's all right, really') or over-dramatic. Almost certainly your symptoms will be familiar to the doctors, and they just need an indication of how much discomfort you are in. Also, use ordinary, everyday language: don't try to adopt the doctors' medical words, which you may not fully understand. They will understand what you are telling them. Just because they sometimes sound as though they are speaking a foreign language, doesn't mean that they don't understand plain English! If you try to pick up and use the medical terminology for your condition you may open up lots of possibilities for misunderstanding.

Your family doctor is always your first point of contact. He or she should be able to talk to you about your cancer and the possible treatments you may have, and then refer you to the appropriate clinic or hospital. The next contact is usually the hospital doctor or specialist: an oncologist is a cancer specialist, and you can ask to be referred to one. You may also wish to be referred to a specialist for the part of the body where the cancer is located. The more specialised the doctor or nurse is, the more they are likely to know about all the details of your symptoms and your likely reactions to treatment. Use their experience to get the best out of the system.

You want to know all the facts – but try not to allow the doom and gloom to get to you. When Roy was first diagnosed he asked our GP to tell him all the facts with no glossing over the hard bits. He did as he was asked – poor man – and said, 'I'd like to tell you that you'll still be here next year, but I can't.' When he had gone, we laughed, simply because the picture he painted was so awful. I said to Roy, 'If I were you, I'd just get on and die now, and save yourself all the trouble!' Yet it was this, I think, that spurred Roy on to defy the illness. He had a lot of things he wanted to do, and he wasn't going to be beaten so easily. He never regretted the time spent in treatment, which won him so much extra, valuable time with his family and friends, and enabled him to achieve so much for other cancer patients.

Your family

Your family, if you have one, can be an immense source of support and comfort. There can be difficulties if yours is not the sort of family which communicates easily, but it is important for your own welfare that you are able to talk about what is happening to you. Repressing your worries and bottling up your feelings will probably make you feel worse. Somehow just expressing your fears can make them seem more manageable, especially if the person you are talking to stays with you and does not react with horror.

Some cancer patients fear that other family members will not be able to cope with discussing the details of their illness. If you are tempted to think like this, try to remember that the illness is happening to you – not to them. You have enough to deal with, being strong for yourself. In any case, this fear is usually unfounded: people do cope and discover unexpected strength. Trying to keep your condition a secret from your family makes life very difficult for the nurses and any others who do know about it – and you really cannot ask people to lie to your family on your behalf. More than anything else, this kind of deception destroys trust, and makes communication even harder.

One woman patient had refused to allow anyone to tell her husband that she was suffering from cancer. However, she was troubled by a recurring dream in which her husband seemed to her to be getting smaller and smaller, and further and further away from her. The dream stopped after she had plucked up the courage to tell a nurse about it, but it seemed clear that in her subconscious her lack of honesty was coming between them at a time when they would probably both have benefited from closeness and trust.

A diagnosis of cancer often makes a strong relationship even stronger, but it is true that it may expose the weakness of a poor relationship. If you are truly afraid to tell your partner or friend, ask yourself what is the worst that can happen? If someone leaves a relationship because they cannot face being near you through an illness, would you really want to deceive them into staying? And for how long would the deception last in any case? Many nurses are skilled in helping friends and relatives discuss their fears, which may often prove to be groundless.

The love and affection of your partner can make a real difference to your general feeling of well-being. Incidentally, there is no medical reason to stop making love because you have cancer, and the sense of comfort, closeness and sharing it generates can be a real help. On the other hand, you may sometimes feel too ill for lovemaking, or anxiety or depression may make you less enthusiastic. Some drug regimes also affect your ability to make love. Your partner may avoid sex out of fear, or be afraid of hurting you or appearing demanding, just when you most need a caress to reassure you that you have not suddenly become unattractive. Whatever the reasons, it is always better if you can manage to talk about the problems; there are many ways of being close and giving comfort in a loving relationship.

Often the other members of the family are unsure how to react. They need some signal from you to know whether you want to talk or not, but once they know, they are usually willing to be as supportive as they can – either by listening, or helping to find out the facts, or at times, if you choose, by ignoring it entirely. One patient said, 'Am I becoming a cancer bore?' If this is one of your fears, then you may need to widen the net of your support system: spread the load among your other friends!

Friends

Just because you have cancer, that does not turn you overnight into a professional patient. Even though there are days when having cancer seems like a full-time job, there will also be days when you want and need to forget about it. You still have the same capacity for fun, enjoyment, entertainment, conversation, and all your other interests: you are still the same person that you were last week, before the diagnosis.

It is true that you may be rather more emotionally fragile than usual, and you may sometimes be physically unable to do things that you used to do, but that does not cancel out your usual interests. You may not play football for a while, but you can still watch a game and debate the quality of the referee's eyesight! You may not feel up to shopping for clothes for yourself, but you can still have an opinion about the latest fashions, or advise your daughter about her choice of make-up.

Your friends can be part of your support system, and that does not necessarily mean that they have to take a course in cancer care. There may be some in whom you confide, and who will be willing to listen to your feelings and fears, but you can be helped just as much by work colleagues who ring up to tell you what is going on at the office, or friends at the pub who may not know you are ill at all.

You probably don't want to become 'a cancer bore', and the best way is to make sure that you have as big a support group as possible. It may sound rather calculating to start working out what your friends can do for you, but this isn't selfish – it's just a case of making the best of a crisis situation. Identify who your support group are, and what you need from them. For instance, who are the friends you can be most honest with, and the ones who know you best?

- Who can you go to when you need a good cry, and know there'll be a box of tissues, a cup of tea, a sympathetic ear, and perhaps a cheering-up laugh afterwards?

- Who will keep you up to date on developments at work when you've been away?
- Who shares your interest in football (or gardening, or whatever your hobbies are)?
- Who has known you a long time, and can remember old times with you?
- Who is always willing to give practical help, mowing the lawn, doing the ironing or getting the shopping?
- Who is good at helping you to think things through and make rational decisions?
- Who has had experience of coping with cancer and knows what the treatment will involve?
- Who will take you out for a good time and not even mention the word cancer?
- Who can help you sort out your finances?
- Who do you know who isn't embarrassed by talking about spiritual things, like praying or life after death?
- Who helps you to feel cheerful and positive, and always makes you laugh?
- Who will tell you all the latest gossip?

It's worth trying to draw up a list like this, because it ensures that you spread the load. You won't keep crying on the same shoulders, and you won't make people feel that all they must talk about in your presence is your cancer (boring for you, as well as for them).

Privately, you might want to draw up a brief list of a non-support group, too: those few individuals who always seem to leave you feeling depressed and exhausted, or want to tell you their troubles. This is not the time to be charitable and put up with them – being ill gives you an excuse to avoid them. Your job is to conserve your energy, not let it be drained by people who want to lean on you. When Roy was ill we received a long letter from a lady who enumerated all her various friends and relatives who had suffered from a wide range of cancers, finishing triumphantly, 'and they all died'! We laughed about this because it was so obviously unhelpful, but it is the sort of thing you are perfectly justified in avoiding.

Counselling

However, not everyone has a wide circle of family and friends to form a support group. Whom do you talk to if you live alone, or indeed, if you really feel you don't want to talk to your friends about your illness? Professional counsellors are people who have been trained to listen, but not to give advice. They are supportive but also objective, and with their skilled questioning and prompting, they can help you to look more clearly at the things which are troubling you. They will not suggest solutions but they can help you to arrive at your own, and because they are not directly involved in your life, they can often enable you to take a cooler look at all the possibilities.

Counselling has proved to be so valuable to many patients that many hospitals now provide their own counselling service, and your GP or hospital may be able to put you in touch with a trained counsellor. The British Association for Counselling can also provide a list of counsellors by region.

Patient groups

There is one group of people who probably understand very well what you are going through, without being told: other patients. When you are attending hospital for treatment visits or for check ups, you meet other people in the waiting room who are there for the same thing. Often a kind of camaraderie develops, as little conversations spring up – perhaps about the waiting time to start with, or the weather, and then going on to talk about the treatment, how many visits you have made, how well or ill you feel. Here at last is a set of people who are not afraid to talk about cancer, and it can be a relief.

Roy was one of those people who always struck up a conversation wherever he was – waiting at a bus stop or standing in a queue at the greengrocer. He was always quick to make a joke, too, so the waiting room at the hospital he attended for his radiotherapy sessions was full of laughter as he clowned about. He was a real showman, and however he was feeling, he always rose to the bait of a captive audience! One of the regulars at this session was a few weeks ahead of him with his treatment, and came to the end of the course first.

'My last treatment today,' he said. 'Do you think they'll mind if I come back next week anyway? I'll miss the show!'

He may have been joking, but underneath he was serious; not just about missing Roy's cheerful good humour, but about missing out on the 'team spirit' which had developed over the weeks in that waiting room. Grumbling and sympathising and laughing together, that particular group of patients gained something from each others' company.

This is why many hospitals now organise patient support groups, particularly for those whose treatment has come to an end. Once your treatment has finished, you may be immensely relieved that it is over, but you may also miss the companionship of other patients. No one can understand your feelings so well as someone who has gone through the same experience. No one can convince you that you will feel better in a month's time, so well as someone who is that much further down the line. And only someone who has stood in the same position as you, can really say, 'Of course you aren't silly to feel like that. I did too.'

At a support group you don't just compare notes on how ill you feel. You may pick up some really useful tips on how to cope with side-effects of treatment (for instance, I learned to liquidise food for Roy when he suffered from mouth ulcers, so that he didn't have to chew). And you can discuss things that you hesitate to talk about with your family or friends, because you know it would upset them. Having a place to go to for all these things can be a real help. Patient.co.uk gives a list of UK sources of information and support, and some of these may be able to put you in touch with groups in your area.

Information

The one word which keeps being repeated here is 'information'. I don't want to give anyone the impression that to get over cancer successfully you are going to need a medical degree! However, once you know that you have this illness you probably want to give yourself the best chance you can. That may mean making sensible decisions when you are offered choices. Do you want to be treated at your local hospital or a specialist one? Do you want to be given the address of your support group? Or even, What do you want to eat? To make the best decision for you means knowing something about the illness and the best ways of dealing with it.

On the other hand, you have to know yourself, and get the right amount of information for your needs. Some people are quite happy to trust the doctors to help them through everything, and really don't want any more information than the absolute minimum. If reading books about cancer is going to depress you, then don't do it! In particular, if you do read anything about medical matters, take note of when it was published: cancer research is moving on rapidly, and treatments change and develop. An out-of-date book may be misleading.

However, most people find that knowledge helps them, just as being around the medical staff in hospital can be comforting. There cancer is not feared and dreaded, but is treated in a matter-of-fact way as an everyday occurrence. An attitude of 'These are the facts, and this is what we are doing about them' can be very reassuring.

So where do you get information? We have already said that the doctors and nurses are your first resource. Next, you might want something in print, that you can take away with you. Books and leaflets can be of two kinds: some, like this book, talk about cancer in general, as though it were one illness. Others are more specialist, and deal with individual specific cancers. The same is true of the various charities and organisations, which may be formed primarily to further research into cancer or to support patients. Some deal with cancer in general and can give you information on a whole range of cancers, while others have a particular interest in one form of cancer. Again.patient.co.uk – whose materials are often printed off by GPs to hand to patients – will direct you to helpful organisations.

Part II

Moving On

Cancer touches every part of your life – not only the physical aspects but also the emotional and spiritual. It is not an experience I would have chosen and I wish I could have learned the life lessons some other gentler way, but through my experience I have come to appreciate the gift of life so much more. I don't take it for granted.

I try to live one day at a time.

It has given me a focus as to what is important in life.

It has opened new doors to me and introduced me to new people.

It has shown me the importance of true friendships.

It has strengthened my faith in God.

Elvira Lowe

4. Working Together

Once you have taken on board all the facts and information about cancer, it is time to move on. Your doctors will no doubt be anxious to start your treatment as soon as possible, to give it the best possible chance of success. You will be keen to work together with the doctors, and to co-operate with whatever they ask of you, but you may be anxious about what is likely to happen next.

Even after you were told that you had cancer, you were probably asked to agree to some further tests. These were designed to find out as much as possible about the type of cancer you have, and what stage and grade it is.

'Staging' establishes how far the cancer has spread: it may be just a single tumour or lump, and it may still be very small, or it may have grown quite large. Some cells may have broken off from it and begun to spread; they may have reached the lymph nodes, which drain the lymph system in your body. Or they may have spread even further, via the lymphatic system or the bloodstream, and have set up some secondary sites (or 'metastases') where new tumours have begun to grow.

'Grading' determines how aggressive the cancer is, and tells the doctors about the degree of malignancy. A low-grade cancer is one which shows few cells dividing and comparatively slow growth; a high-grade cancer shows very abnormal cells and very rapid growth. One compensation is that the high-grade cancers often respond more quickly to treatment.

The results of these tests will have helped the doctors to decide on how to treat your cancer. There are three main groups of treatment at the moment: surgery, radiotherapy and drugs (chemotherapy or hormone therapy). Any one or a combination of these may be used.

You will be asked to sign a consent form agreeing to any of these treatments. You should sign this only when you are clear in your own mind about what is going to happen, why the treatment is offered, what it hopes to achieve, what the side-effects may be, and whether you are happy to have it.

Surgery

Surgery means an operation in which you will be given a general anaesthetic so that you are very deeply unconscious. This enables the surgeon to cut away the abnormal tissue. A single tumour in one location may be suitable for surgery (and indeed, you may have already had a tiny sample of the tumour removed for diagnosis). Although surgery may remove the bulk of a tumour, it is not possible to distinguish cancer cells with the naked eye, so in some cases it is unlikely that the surgeon will be able to take away every last abnormal cell. Those cells remaining in the body will go on multiplying unless they are removed or killed: this is why surgery is often followed by chemotherapy or radiotherapy, to mop up any straggling cells left behind.

Radiotherapy

Radiotherapy uses high-energy rays to destroy cancer cells. You probably know that it is quite safe to have an x-ray which is used to look inside your body (for instance to examine a broken bone), but that too many x-rays or too large a dose can be dangerous, because these rays damage cells. Many types of cancer cells are more sensitive to these rays than normal cells, and radiotherapy exploits this by using a very carefully measured dose: large enough to damage the cancer cells, but not large enough to cause serious harm to healthy cells.

Radiotherapy may be used on its own to destroy a tumour, or to shrink it to make the patient more comfortable (for instance, if the tumour is pressing on another organ). It may be used before surgery to make a tumour smaller and easier to remove, or after surgery to kill off any remaining cancer cells.

The dose has to be carefully assessed, and it is usually divided into a series of treatments to be delivered over a period of days or weeks. There is usually a planning session, when the area to be targeted is marked with purple dye or a series of dots, and then the patient is placed in position and the machine is lined up. The radiotherapist then leaves the area. This is not because the procedure is particularly dangerous at any one session, but a radiotherapist working in this environment all day, every day, has to be very careful not to receive lots of tiny doses of radiation accidentally, which could add up to a dose large enough to be harmful. It may feel rather alarming to be left alone with a large machine like this, but the therapy usually lasts only a few minutes.

Chemotherapy

Chemotherapy is treatment with drugs which destroy cancer cells, usually when they are in the process of dividing. Often a mixture of drugs will be used, with each drug having a slightly different effect on the cells: the doctors will make extensive inquiries to try to determine the right drug 'cocktail' for you. Hospitals have access to an extensive database of information about different cancers, drugs and patients, so that they are often able to say with reasonable accuracy that for a patient of your age with your symptoms a certain combination of drugs is likely to be the most effective.

Small doses may be in pill form, but usually the drugs are administered by injection or drip. When they have to be delivered slowly over a period of hours, this may involve a stay overnight in hospital. Because the drugs circulate around your body through your bloodstream, they affect all your cells. Like radiotherapy, chemotherapy relies on the fact that the cancer cells are more vulnerable than your healthy cells; however, a single treatment is seldom enough to kill off the cancer cells, so the treatment has to be repeated. Since your normal cells will recover faster than the cancer cells, a short period of rest is allowed between treatments. The idea is to cause progressive damage to the cancer cells, while allowing the normal cells to recuperate.

Improvements in drug therapy are being introduced all the time, reducing the need for radical surgery. Because chemotherapy cannot be targeted at one area of the body, but affects all cells, you are more likely to experience side-effects from this treatment, but improvements are also being made to other drugs which help to counteract these effects.

Other treatments

There are several other treatments which may be possible for you. Hormones are chemical substances which are produced naturally by the body, and control reproduction and other functions; hormone therapy can be used for cancers of the breast, prostate, thyroid and uterus.

Bone marrow is the spongy inner part of large bones where blood cells are made: occasionally bone marrow may be extracted from a healthy (and suitable) donor and transplanted into a cancer patient to replace this function after radiotherapy or chemotherapy has damaged it. Sometimes a similar activity can be performed by peripheral blood stem transplants, in which stem cells can be collected from the patient's own blood, and then put back later into the bloodstream.

The rate at which cancer care is advancing is encouraging. New treatments are being devised all the time: current developments include vaccines and gene therapy. If current treatments can keep people alive for a few years, then the new treatments which are now on the horizon may be able to give them further extra years, if not a cure. Research is offering patients real hope.

What do I need to know?

You can see from all the above that cancer treatments are designed to kill off cells that are already cancerous. In spite of all the rapid advances being made in research, we still do not know how to prevent cancer, nor how to detect it at its very earliest stages, when the system of cell division starts to go wrong. Because of this, the treatment which kills the unhealthy cancer cells is likely to damage some of your normal, healthy cells as well, and that will probably make you feel unwell. However, a few months of discomfort can be the gateway to many years of healthy, active life.

When Victoria Kagi faced her bone marrow transplant, the doctor warned her that the treatment was going to be 'like crossing the North Pole'. In total it took several months, including chemotherapy, radiation therapy and a period in isolation while her own immune system recovered; however, she reported that she made a good recovery afterwards, 'getting slowly but surely stronger every day, with the help of my family and lots of rest, exercise and physiotherapy ... it was worth it.'

Most cancer treatments make demands on the patient, especially if you were not feeling particularly ill at the time when you were diagnosed: it seems hard that the treatment should make you feel worse! The following sections deal with some of the side-effects you may experience from your treatment, but it is important to remember that not everyone suffers the same effects, or to the same extent. Everyone's body is different, and responds differently to these very finely graded dosages. You should always tell your nurse about any symptom, to check that it really is a result of your treatment. A minute on the phone could save you a month of worry.

So why should you find out anything in advance about possible side-effects? Won't it just worry you? There are two answers to this. Firstly, it often helps to be prepared: digestive trouble, or hair loss, or anything else, is less alarming if you are forewarned. Secondly, if you should experience something out of the ordinary, you are more likely to query it with the doctors if you have some idea of what the expected effects are likely to be.

Betty Napper was treated for ovarian cancer nearly twenty years ago; after surgery, she had monthly chemotherapy sessions for six months. 'The chemo wasn't too bad,' she says, 'except for the first one. I felt terrible – I kept fidgeting and couldn't sit still. I kept standing up and sitting down again, and then I started to shake all over. I knew that couldn't be right. No one had said that would happen. We called the doctor, and he gave me something to stop it – sort of switch it off. After that they changed the dose and everything was fine. My hair fell out a little bit, but I've got thick hair and so it didn't show. I didn't need a wig!'

Questions to ask

The list below includes some of the questions you might want to ask your doctor or nurse before your treatment starts.

- What treatments are available? What choice do I have?
- What is this treatment for – to cure the disease, to help me live longer or to deal with my symptoms?

- What benefits do you expect from the treatment?
- What does the treatment involve?
- How long will the treatment go on for? How long will each session be?
- Where will I have to go for treatment? Will I need to stay in hospital or attend as an out-patient?
- Will I be able to come and go from hospital alone, or will I need someone with me?
- Will I be allowed to drive?
- Will I need time off work?
- What will be the immediate side-effects?
- Will there be any longer-term effects?
- Will the treatment affect my sex life?
- Will I need to change what I eat?
- What effects should I watch out for, that might need to be reported to a doctor?

Possible side-effects of cancer treatments

Some side-effects are the same in several kinds of cancer therapies – for instance, tiredness, nausea and skin irritation can follow both radiation therapy and chemotherapy – so it is simpler here to point out just a few of the more common side-effects, rather than trying to be exhaustive about each treatment. You should ask for information leaflets about your particular treatment or consult one of the specific cancer websites for more detailed information. Remember that some people experience very few of these effects, and that many of them can be effectively controlled by medication.

Anxiety

It is difficult to know whether anxiety and depression are caused by the treatment or by the simple fact of having cancer, but both are very common. Both can be helped by a variety of approaches, ranging from medication to counselling, but should always be reported to your doctor or nurse. You need all your mental and physical reserves to tackle your treatment, and feeling low, irritable and weepy only wears you out.

Fatigue

Fatigue, on the other hand, is a well recognised side-effect of all the main treatments. After surgery you are likely to feel tired as your body recovers from the operation and builds scar tissue. Tiredness and lethargy are common after both radiotherapy and chemotherapy, too, sometimes for months after the treatment. It is important to allow yourself plenty of time to recover, and not to make too many demands on yourself too soon.

Self-image

Depression, worry and emotional problems can also result from changes in your feelings about yourself and your body. If your body changes – perhaps because you have lost or gained weight, or because of the visible effects of surgery – you feel differently about yourself. You may be self-conscious because of a mastectomy (when all or part of a breast is removed), or because of wearing a bag after a colostomy for bowel cancer. These changes in your mental image of your own body may depress you, and may also cause you to worry that you are no longer attractive to your partner. Even if the damage to your body is internal and invisible, you may still feel differently about yourself.

It can be difficult to come to terms with these changes in your life, but they are a price that most people are willing to pay in order to win their fight with cancer. Sorting out your feelings may take time, but it is possible to learn to live with the changes, especially if you have a supportive family and partner. You know that you do not love your family because of their appearance: each person is much more important than that, and you would not stop loving someone if they lost an arm or a leg in an accident. Similarly, they are unlikely to reject you because of what has happened; they are probably only too relieved that you are still with them.

Lymphoedema

Lymphoedema is a swelling – usually of an arm or leg – caused by cancer or by its treatment. It happens when a lymph channel is blocked, either by a tumour or by scarring from radiotherapy or surgery. The lymph fluid is unable to drain away through the usual channels, and so it builds up and seeps into the surrounding tissues, making the limb feel swollen, heavy and difficult to move. There is a great deal that can be done to treat this condition, including skin care, compression sleeves and stockings, and physiotherapy, exercise and massage.

Urinary problems

Several chemotherapy drugs affect the kidneys and bladder, causing urgency (you may be unable to wait), pain and burning when you urinate, red or orange colour in the urine, strange smelling urine, or fever. You should always check that these symptoms are caused by your medication, and not by any other infection.

Skin irritation

Radiotherapy can have an effect like sunburn on the skin: it may become dry and sore or itchy. Chemotherapy also may make the skin dry and more sensitive to sunlight: you should avoid putting any deodorants, ointments or perfume on the skin, other than prescribed creams or sunblock. Avoid extreme temperatures (no hot baths), and do not scrub it. Wear soft, loose clothing over any affected areas.

Mouth problems

The cells of the mouth lining divide very rapidly, so they are very likely to be damaged by chemotherapy aimed at dividing cells. Mouth soreness or ulcers are common, which can make eating difficult. It is still important to take care of your teeth and gums, however, so you should try to clean your teeth with a very soft brush or even with a mouth swab after every meal. If toothpaste is too strong, you could rinse with bicarbonate of soda dissolved in warm water. Very soft foods with lots of added liquid are easier to swallow, and you should avoid highly spiced, salty or acid foods (like vinegar, pickles or lemon) which will make things worse. You may be prescribed ointments and mouthwashes to help.

Digestive problems

Loss of appetite and nausea are common after both radiotherapy (especially when the treated area is near the stomach) and chemotherapy (because the digestive system is another area where normal cells are dividing rapidly). There are many very effective anti-nausea drugs available which can be prescribed to control this, provided you tell the doctor what is happening to you and do not suffer in silence. You can also help yourself by avoiding very hot, strong-smelling foods (cold foods may be more palatable at this time), and by eating small amounts of food more often. It is frustrating to feel unable to eat, when you know you need to keep your strength up: take plenty of liquids, and aim for high-protein, soft, and even liquidised meals if necessary.

If you suffer from diarrhoea, forget the usual advice about healthy fruit and high-fibre diets. Drink plenty of fluids but avoid too much milk, and eat small meals more often, including fish or chicken, eggs and white bread, pasta and rice.

Hair loss

Hair grows from its roots in your scalp, and hair roots are another place likely to be damaged by some forms of chemotherapy. After a couple of weeks of treatment, your hair may begin to fall out. Different drugs have different effects, so the degree to which this happens can vary, but it is still a shock to find your hair falling out on the pillow or in your hairbrush, or when you wash it. Fortunately this is a temporary condition, and you can expect your hair to grow back once the treatment is over, though it may be a different colour, or either curlier or straighter than before.

Nevertheless some people, especially women, find this very distressing, on a par with other changes to their self-image. Jeannette Barwick says that the thought which woke her in the night with a sense of panic was 'Would I lose my hair? I realised I could die from this cancer, but the panic came over my hair!' On the other hand, Roy cheerfully shaved off his few remaining wisps and went around with his bald head held high. He was greatly helped by our good friend Don Maclean who said he thought his bald head was brilliant: 'It means you can go to fancy-dress parties dressed as a roll-on deodorant!' Not everyone can be so cheerful about it. If you decide that a wig will make you feel less self-conscious, it is a good idea to have a fitting before you have lost all your own hair, to match your natural colour better. Some people prefer to experiment with scarves or hats.

Damage to blood cells

Another area affected by chemotherapy is the bone marrow. The blood cells made in the spongy area inside our large bones are of three types. First there are the red blood cells, which carry oxygen around the body; then there are the white blood cells, which help to fight the viruses and bacteria which cause infections; and finally the platelets, which help our blood to clot. When these cells are damaged, a variety of symptoms result: that is why you have to have so many blood tests during chemotherapy, so that the doctors can keep a close eye on exactly what effect the treatment is having on your healthy cells.

When red blood cells are damaged, your blood is less able to carry oxygen around the body, so your muscles are starved of oxygen. You may feel dizzy, weak, tired or breathless. The remedy is to take plenty of rest, and wait until your natural red blood count recovers before having more treatment. You may need a transfusion of someone else's healthy blood to build you up again.

When white blood cells are damaged, your ability to fight off infections is reduced. These cells divide rapidly, so they repair themselves quickly, too, but in the meantime you need to avoid crowded places where you might more easily pick up coughs and colds. It is important to be especially careful with personal hygiene, and to report to the doctor at once if you notice any of the usual signs of infection (such as a high temperature, cough or sore throat, vaginal soreness, pain on urination, tenderness around a wound, etc.).

When the platelet count in your blood drops too low, your blood does not clot as well as usual. This means that you may bruise easily, and if you accidentally cut or graze your skin you may bleed much more heavily than usual. Take extra care with dental floss or when brushing teeth, and with scissors, needles, tools and so on.

Dealing with symptoms

These are by no means all the possible side-effects that can occur, but you should bear in mind that neither will you suffer from all of them. Some patients feel very angry if they suffer from a side-effect of their treatment which they have not been warned about, but others can feel very depressed just at the thought of all the possible things that can happen to them. It is hard for doctors to steer a course between everyone's different requirements. The important thing is to make a note of any symptom that worries or distresses you, and check up with your nurse or doctor: it may not be anything to do with your cancer treatment, but be something quite different which needs dealing with in a different way. Even if it is caused by your treatment, there may still be many ways of overcoming it or treating it.

Lynn Faulds Wood says,

> I found that trying to get control over my life was a good coping mechanism. Insomnia is common with people who are told they have cancer. I took sleeping pills for the first month and then tried hypnotherapy to cure it. Getting up and watching TV in the middle of the night until I felt sleepy again turned out to be the best solution for me.

> After a few months, I developed a bad back, lifting my three-year-old son. Bad backs are common with people who have had stomach surgery – and I had the full zipper from beneath my breast bone to the top of my pelvic area. I found acupuncture fantastic for easing the worst of my bad back. Massage oil (with a few drops of patchouli oil in it to promote healing) helped soften the scar and today it is barely visible.

> The best advice I had was the warning that having cancer is an emotional roller-coaster, with up days and down days. Once I was able to get about, a brisk walk helped to life my spirits on the low days.

When Roy was going through his treatment, he visited lots of patients on cancer wards. He used to say, 'Don't forget, however bad the treatment makes you feel, it's making the cancer feel worse!'

Clinical trials

Researchers are always trying to improve the methods of treatment for cancer. To do that they first have to work out a theory of what might work, then develop it, and then try it out and see how well it compares with current treatments. Before any new drug or therapy reaches the stage of clinical trials (that is, on real patients), it will already have been tested in a variety of ways to show that it is safe – indeed, some trials are conducted merely to identify the best dosage or method of delivery (pill, injection, etc) for a drug whose effects are already proven.

Trials have to be fair – that means that the patients involved have to be randomly chosen. This ensures that there can be no weighting of the results: no doctor can choose to give a new drug only to patients with slow-growing, early-stage cancer, who would be expected to do well anyway. This would make it appear that the particular drug was specially effective.

Trials are usually conducted with one group of patients using the new drug or delivery system, and another similar group (the 'control' group) using the standard treatment. If you agree to take part, you will not be told which group you are in. However, if (as occasionally happens) the new treatment is quickly shown to be benefiting patients enormously, then the trial will be stopped and everyone who is suitable will be offered the better treatment.

You are able to choose freely whether to participate in clinical trials; your treatment will be no better or worse whatever you decide. (At the very least you will be receiving the standard treatment, which will be the best and most effective currently on offer.) You will be asked to complete a detailed consent form and given a copy to keep. All clinical trials are rigorously controlled by local and national ethics committees, to ensure that you are told exactly what is involved, and that no undue pressure is placed upon patients or unrealistic promises made to them.

You can also pull out of the trial if you decide that you don't want to continue any longer. Your doctor will provide another treatment for you.

If you decide to take part, you will be making a real contribution to the fight against cancer.

5. Living with Cancer

When we talk about cancer, its diagnosis and its treatment, it is easy to concentrate on the technicalities. We talk about what is happening at the level of individual cells, or what certain chemical processes involve. All this is very important, and we are certainly grateful to the scientists and doctors whose research enables them to understand the disease at this cellular level: it is their findings which develop the treatments which can cure or hold back the illness. However, at the same time, thinking about the disease in terms of cells and treatments can be misleading. It seems to encourage us to think about it as something that is happening to our body, as though that could somehow be separate from what happens to our mind.

The fact is that our minds and our bodies are inextricably linked, in ways which no one properly understands yet. It is true that your mood may be altered by some of the chemical effects of the drugs, but also your feelings may change from day to day, as a result of the emotional effects of the whole experience of having cancer. Whatever stage you are at – newly diagnosed, having treatment, recovering, or even if your cancer is long in the past – you may still find that you experience unusual emotions.

Even people whose cancer is in remission often go on feeling changed and disturbed by the experience. Elizabeth Harrison had extensive surgery for bowel cancer. She says, 'I always thought of myself as a strong person, a slayer of dragons! I fought for what I believed in. Now my cancer has been dealt with, and it's in the past, but it has left me feeling different. Now I feel so vulnerable. Once you have to confront your own mortality like that, it changes you.'

Some people fear that their cancer will come back, and this haunts them so much that they can't get on with living their life. Others suffer a whole range of emotional upheavals which worry them. Yet others manage to cope with their own feelings, but are confused by the reactions they get from their friends and family. What kind of feelings do people report, and what causes them?

Being in control

When you are well, you can choose your own activities, how you spend your time and who you spend it with. Once you are ill, you lose some of this freedom. You may be unable to do many of the things you normally enjoy; you may have to be cared for in hospital, and put up with uncomfortable treatment. You realise that you cannot control your own health – you have contracted this disease unknowingly and unwillingly. You may have chosen to accept treatment because you want to get better, but that does not make it any easier to accept the pressures of hospital routines, or the waiting around at clinics which make demands on your time.

The whole experience may make you feel that you are no longer in charge of your life, and that control has passed to the doctors and nurses, and even to the staff who bring you your meals in hospital! People react to this in various ways. Some people seem to switch onto a sort of auto-pilot: they become passive, accepting whatever they are told but asking no questions and taking little active interest in their own condition. They take everything one step at a time, and refuse to look ahead. This is a very common reaction, especially during a period of intensive treatment or during a stay in hospital. Family and friends may find it strange if you have normally been a very active, involved person, but this can be a very healthy reaction. You may be instinctively giving yourself time to cope and take in what is happening, at a time when it is safe to give up control to those who are caring for you.

Most people then move on from this initial stage, beginning to take an interest in their treatment and in what will happen next. The more they talk to doctors and nurses about what is involved in their care, the more they begin to feel in control. There are choices and decisions to be made, and they are able to make them.

Often they also begin to look for things which will help them personally to feel better – such as exercise, or some activity which takes their mind off things – and that also helps them to feel more in control of their own lives.

The stages of grief

Coming to terms with the fact that you have cancer can take time, and it has been likened to the developing process that people go through when someone close to them dies. In a way, there has been a death, because you have lost part of yourself: your old, healthy self. You may feel that you have also lost a lot of other things. You may have lost part of your role as a strong healthy father figure who could support a family, or as a capable mother who provided meals and ran the home. You may have lost your role in the office or factory as a good, reliable worker, or as the friend other people depended on. You may feel that you have lost your interest in planning for the future, which may now look frighteningly uncertain.

For all these reasons, having a serious illness is very like being bereaved, and you may experience many of the same emotions that are common to the process of grieving for someone or something you have lost. There are recognised stages in this process.

First there may be denial: 'It can't be true,' or 'This can't be happening to me.' The kind of denial mentioned in Chapter 1, at the time of diagnosis, can go on for a while. After this you may become angry, and say 'Why me?' (Roy always said, 'Why not me? I'm no different from anyone else!') People who never think about God for five minutes when they are well, suddenly decide that he exists and that it's his fault for allowing this happen to them, and get angry with him as well. (Again, Roy said that he didn't expect God to shield him specially from any of the things that happen to everyone else, including cancer; but he did trust God to help him to get through it.)

Next may come a period of depression, or mourning, when you begin to accept that life really has changed and that you have to go through the process of this illness, whatever the outcome at the end. Finally, you arrive at acceptance. This does not mean that you go back to being passive and just being resigned to whatever happens next. Rather, it means that you have accepted the reality of what is happening, and you take an active part in that, planning for the future, making decisions, and adapting readily to new situations.

The fact that your emotions change and develop like this can be very difficult for your family and friends, especially as they are probably going through the same process, though not necessarily at the same speed. It may seem to them and to you that as soon as you have got used to people behaving in one way, they start changing and feeling different. It all means that talking to one another, being honest about your feelings and explaining what you are thinking, is very important. You have to stay in touch if you are to get through this difficult time without having blazing rows or feeling miserable and rejected and confused.

Negative feelings

It is true that there are strong links between body and mind, and that we do not fully understand the effects one can have on the other. However, some people have been unduly influenced by the school of thought that suggests that 'positive thinking' can help your recovery, and they have interpreted this to mean that having negative feelings will make it harder for you to get well.

This adds yet another burden to the poor patient's back: now not only do you feel miserable because you are ill, but you feel guilty because being depressed may be making you worse! The only sensible course is to accept that you are going to feel miserable at times – you would hardly be normal if you didn't – and that there is no reason to blame yourself for this. At the same time it is as well to look at some of these negative feelings and come to terms with them, and make sure that you don't get so caught up in them that you can't get out.

A typical example is the tendency to blame yourself: for instance, for smoking for many years before developing lung cancer. This makes the illness even harder to bear, if you feel that you have brought it on yourself. Yet no one does such a thing intentionally, and you need to find ways to accept it, forgive yourself and move on. Virtually everyone who develops lung cancer after years of smoking deeply regrets their habit; yet they may have tried to give it up many times, but been unable to do so because of the strongly addictive properties of nicotine. The fault lies with the cigarette: there is nothing to be gained now by agonising over your supposed 'guilt'.

In the same way it is normal to feel angry, but if you keep going round on the same treadmill of thoughts ('Why didn't the doctor investigate sooner? Why didn't the nurse warn me about this side-effect?) you wear yourself out. Sometimes just telling someone how angry you feel can be a relief, as long as you don't make it an opportunity to go through the whole thing again.

Some people live with the constant fear that their cancer will come back, even after they have finished their treatment. Or they have a whole series of fears about pain, or losing their job, or losing the love of their families, which they feel always in the background of their lives. Once again, the only way to deal with such things is to do as much as possible to set your mind at rest (perhaps by talking about pain relief to the nurse, checking up with the human resources officer at work, or sharing your fears with your partner), and then doing your best to put them on one side. Such fears, anger and other feelings can add to the natural stress of being ill, and stress can be exhausting. All of these things together can tip you over into real depression, another added burden at a difficult time.

The best advice, in summary, is to look all these negative feelings in the face. Try to work out what exactly you are worried about, and do your best to do something positive about it. You can get rid of a lot of stress by exercise or by relaxation, and you can sort out a great deal of your fear and anger by talking things through with an understanding friend or a counsellor. Then try to put them behind you so that you are free to concentrate on getting well and on living your own life, day by day.

Time for yourself

Having cancer can be a very lonely experience: however many caring and loving people surround you, in the end the illness is happening in your body, not theirs, and only you know what it feels like. Some people feel devastated by this aloneness. Others, however, find it opens up new attitudes and freedoms. Many people spend most of their lives taking others into account – their parents, children, partner or friends. This new awareness of yourself can make you take note of what you want for the first time for years. You may start doing things that you enjoy, simply because the burden of doing things that you 'ought' to do has been eased by being ill.

Sometimes you may find that you need to be alone, in order to come to terms with all this, and learn to accept fully this business of being aware of yourself as an individual. Many people find this a strange and unsettling experience, but they often feel as though they are 'growing' as an individual. Some people see it as a spiritual rather than an emotional change, and find that as they look at themselves as a person in their own right, they also start to wonder what makes them the person they are: are they more than just a body and a mind? Is there a part of you that is truly unique, unaffected by illness, or drugs and treatments? If you do have a soul or spirit which is truly you, how does it relate to your everyday experience of life? Is there a spiritual aspect of life which we usually ignore? In fact, is there a God who watches and waits for us to become aware of him?

Many people don't go through this kind of thinking, but for others it becomes very exciting to find that through this experience they have uncovered a whole aspect of life which they never thought about before.

Through others' eyes

Even while you are learning to deal with your own changing and developing feelings about your illness, you will realise that you still have to deal with the reactions of those around you. Your immediate family and closest friends may mirror your feelings very closely: they may share your shock, denial, anger and grief. Because of this they may not be able to be as supportive as you would like: it's no good having books like this one telling you to talk about your feelings and your illness to your friends, if they are overwhelmed with fear or unhappiness themselves, and cannot bear to talk about it to you.

Sometimes friends or carers are so intimidated by the illness that they cannot face its reality: they may cling to the idea that a mistake has been made in diagnosis, or they may insist on believing that there is nothing to worry about and everything will be all right. Optimism has its place, but it is not helpful if you yourself are wanting to look soberly at all the possibilities. People who keep saying that there is nothing to worry about offer no support to patients who really need to talk through their fears. Some people's phobia about cancer is so extreme that they cannot bring themselves to think about it seriously.

Sometimes these difficult phases pass; if they do not, you may find that there is no point in continuing the discussion. It is not your job to be a counsellor and supporter for others, and you may decide to avoid old friends who cannot cope with the realities which you are facing.

Just as you may suffer from worry or fear, so may your family or carers. They may be busy all day, trying to go to work, run the house, visit you in hospital or care for your needs at home, so that they hardly have time to stop and think. Then they may lie awake at night worrying about how they will go on coping and what will happen in the future. They may feel frustrated because you cannot share the burden of caring for the family, or because your illness has spoiled your shared plans and limited both your lives for a while. They may even be trying to spare you by not telling you how they are feeling. It is easy to imagine the complex web of resentment and irritation that can build up when everyone is under stress like this.

Once again the only real answer is to try to talk about your feelings honestly, understanding that no one is perfect and that it is normal for everyone to feel angry, lonely, depressed or irritated from time to time. Accepting that you are both human and will be bound to make mistakes, get upset or upset each other is part of any relationship. Learning to cope with your own feelings and someone else's is hard, but not impossible.

Who cares for the carers?

Shortly after Roy started his course of treatment for lung cancer, I went down with the worst flu I have ever had; no doubt the worry and stress had lowered my immune system, too. At the same time we were involved in filming for the BBC series 'Fighting Back', about how people coped with their illnesses. Roy had agreed to take part, and so I had to drive the car on one visit to the hospital accompanied by a film crew and all their equipment. I was feeling terrible, but it seemed pathetic to complain about a little virus when Roy was suffering from a life-threatening disease! In fact, at that stage, Roy was still feeling more or less normal and healthy, and he was probably the fitter of the two of us, but I couldn't ask him to look after me! In any case, once his immune system had been depressed by the treatment, I had to move out of the bedroom, and wear a mask when preparing his food, so that I didn't infect him with my germs. It was a difficult time.

On another occasion Roy was feeling very ill from the chemotherapy; he couldn't even lift his head from the pillow, and clearly wasn't going to be well enough to attend a major public event he had been booked for – an 'Aerobathon' at the Earls Court Exhibition Centre in aid of the Royal Marsden Hospital. He always hated to let people down, but the treatment was such that we simply couldn't predict on which days he would be well enough to work.

'Let me ring and cancel tomorrow,' I suggested. 'The organisers will be sure to understand. No one can possibly blame you for not being there.'

To my amazement, Roy sat up in a fury. 'Why can't you leave me alone?' he shouted. 'It's my life and my business. Just don't interfere. Why don't you get out of the house and don't come back!'

I fled downstairs in tears. A few minutes later the phone rang, and it was Roy, ringing from the bedroom to apologise. It had been a totally uncharacteristic outburst, brought on perhaps by his frustration at letting people down, or by irritation at having to let someone else organise his life.

After that I was careful to watch what I said, making it clear that I wasn't trying to take over decisions about how much he could do. I knew that Roy was being careful too, trying not to let irritation overcome him. I can imagine that this sort of situation is repeated in many homes up and down the country where there is a cancer patient and a partner trying to deal with all this. The problem is that both of you are having to adjust constantly to a situation that changes daily.

It is important for carers to give themselves some space, too. It may be that a one-hour visit to the hospital seems very short to the patient, who is cooped up there all day. For the carer, however, it may involve a three-hour round trip, while trying to juggle a job, housework and meals. It has to be acceptable for carers to say that they cannot visit every day, and not feel guilty in their turn for not providing as much support as the patient would like. Roy's twenty-four hours a week at the hospital was the one opportunity for me to shop, get my hair cut, and so on, so I never visited him during that day while he was having his treatment. It may have seemed callous to the nurses, but I desperately needed that time to myself.

Once again, we have to accept that partners and friends are only human. We are bound to get irritated when we come home and find that the sink is full of dishes: even if we do make a snappy or sarcastic remark, it does not mean that we are bad people, only tired, stressed and worried people. If we do snap, though, it's only fair to apologise and try to do better next time. That's the most anyone can ask. Both patient and carers have to accept their own weakness and weariness, and be prepared to forgive one another.

The advice given above to the cancer patient, about finding a support group, applies just as much to the carer. It is important to accept offers of help: when someone says, 'Is there anything I can do?' it may seem easier to say 'No, I'm fine, thanks.' But in fact it is often a kindness to both of you to say, 'Well, I have got this enormous pile of ironing – could you take just a bit of it away?' or perhaps, 'Could you take over the responsibility of contacting this list of people and pass on the latest news? Then I won't have to spend hours on the phone or computer in the evening.' It lightens your burden, and the concerned friend has the pleasure of doing something that really helps.

It is important that the carers take care of themselves and allow others to help: if their physical and emotional energy is too run down, they won't be in a position to help the patient. They, too, need time off from thinking about cancer. They can bear the pain with the patient, but they cannot bear it for them; allowing themselves to suffer and get worn down helps no one.

Achieving a balance

Living with cancer is rather like riding a roller-coaster: every week, every day has its ups and downs. Just when everything seems to be going well, some unforeseen change of mood, or some unexpected symptom plunges you down again. In the same way, when everyone is feeling low, some unexpected bonus, some improvement or new medication can make the world seem a much brighter place, and enable life to go on just as it always did.

Sometimes the hardest thing seems to be to achieve a balance. As the patient improves, so the role of the carer adjusts and reduces: some little task or action which was so much appreciated yesterday is quite unnecessary today. One day the demands on your time seem excessive, the next day you feel rejected and surplus to requirements as the patient feels able to do those things alone. Being aware of all these changes is very demanding, and we all get it wrong sometimes. But many people find that they learn a new sensitivity to their own and each others' moods, and that their whole relationship is enhanced by this way of caring.

6. Helping yourself

It can be comforting to have friends and relations who care about you and who want to help. It is good to know that the doctors and the hospital team are working so hard to speed your recovery from cancer. At the same time, however, you probably want to know if there is anything you can be doing to help yourself, and to improve your chances of recovery. This is when you begin to take note of other people's experiences with the disease, and to look around for other therapies which may help.

As well as all the standard treatments mentioned in earlier chapters, you will doubtless hear about many other possibilities. A whole host of therapies are available, ranging from the common-sense (such as relaxation, massage and diet) to the outrageous (one lady sent a roll of copper wire from Germany for us to wind around our bed, and said that we should make sure it faced in a certain direction if we wanted to be sure that Roy would recover from his cancer). How can you steer your way through all the possibilities on offer?

Whenever you hear about a non-standard treatment (that is, one which is not offered by your doctor or hospital) you should think about it carefully. Such treatments are nearly always recommended to you by well-meaning friends who are anxious to be helpful, and who may be keen to find anything which will improve your condition. Occasionally, however, they may be put forward by people who are trying to make money, and who are willing to take advantage of the vulnerability of the cancer patient. A person who is ill and afraid may well be prepared to grasp at straws, and this can make them easy prey for plausible accounts of magical success stories. Roy was sent many of these because of the publicity his illness engendered; I suppose their owners thought that if he was cured, they would gain both money and fame from their patent 'cure'.

Many therapies are harmless, and may benefit you through increasing your feeling of well-being, or your sense that you are taking an active part in getting well. Others may actually be damaging; the worst ones advocate ignoring the doctors and abandoning proven hospital treatments in favour of untested theories.

The crucial issue is proof: the standard treatments have been subjected to rigorous examination to check that they are effective. Clinical trials will have been conducted, using volunteer patients, to check the range of operation of each drug, the method of delivery, the right dosage, and the possible side effects. Experienced pharmacists will have double-checked the possible interactions between the various drugs and therapies, so that one thing you are taking does not interfere with another. All of this has to happen before a drug can be licensed for use in this country.

The alternatives have very seldom been tested in any scientific way, and their promises of miracle cures are usually anecdotal. You will hear stories about people who have made miraculous recoveries from illness: what such accounts are seldom able to tell you is whether the person was undergoing any other treatment at the time, what else they were taking, or indeed, whether the therapy has been shown to have effects which can be reliably repeated when applied to other patients. One or two successes can be coincidence: it takes a properly conducted scientific trial to prove effectiveness. Dr Robert Buckman investigated many such stories for a television series he was working on. Often the account would appear to be reliable, but when it was carefully and objectively followed up, in some cases by checking medical records, there always proved to be something to throw doubt on the success stories.

Having said this, doctors do admit that there are many things they do not yet fully understand. Homoeopathy, for instance, is a system of medication based on giving patients very dilute amounts of various substances. The dilutions are so great that the quantities of the original substance are scarcely detectable, and there seems to be no reason why they should have any effect on the body. When taken in the prescribed manner they have never been shown to do any harm. Yet for certain conditions homoeopathy can be effective. Some NHS doctors have voluntarily taken training in how to use it, and they offer it to their patients as an additional service. Others believe that the effectiveness is due only to the patient's belief in the medication.

So if you hear about a treatment which is said to help cancer patients, how can you know whether it is either useful or safe?

What kind of treatment?

There are three main kinds of treatment which you may hear about.

The first are standard or conventional therapies. These are the ones we have already discussed at length, such as surgery, radiotherapy and chemotherapy. They are tried and tested, and are used all over the world as the accepted and proven treatments. They have measurable and reliable effects on reducing or curing cancer.

The second type are called complementary therapies. They are often given alongside the conventional treatments for cancer, but they do not claim to cure the disease when used alone. They can, however, be of real benefit in alleviating symptoms and side-effects. Some of them are so well accepted as useful by the medical profession that they are regarded as part of the range of standard support for patients: they include counselling, psychotherapy and relaxation techniques. Others, though not part of conventional support systems, may also be offered at hospitals and treatment centres, such as massage, aromatherapy, self-help groups or art therapy.

The third kind are called alternative therapies, because they claim to cure cancer when they are used instead of the conventional therapies. It is these which concern doctors the most, because their practitioners invariably attempt to use unconventional means to treat the cancer, and insist or suggest that the patient should abandon conventional treatment. Many cancer doctors believe that some of these 'cures' can be harmful or even dangerous, quite apart from the danger of abandoning a proven treatment which may be doing you good.

In your mind

Any strategy that helps you to cope with cancer is likely to be helpful, and there are many techniques aimed at helping you to deal with your own emotional responses and the stress that accompanies any major illness. No one knows whether reducing stress can actually improve the likelihood of your recovery in the future, but there is no doubt that it makes you feel better today. Improving the quality of your everyday life must be a good thing.

Counselling amounts to little more than talking – or rather, listening! – and you can get a great deal of help from the informal talking you do with your family and friends. However, there are sometimes things which you are not willing to discuss with them, or perhaps you do not have anyone close enough to you to confide in. In this case the counsellor's trained listening skills can be useful. Counsellors can help you to express and understand your feelings, without offering you any advice or intrusive accounts of their own experiences, such as usually accompanies ordinary conversations!

Organised self-help groups also rely on the beneficial effects of talking and discussion. They allow patients and their families to meet others who are in the same situation, and provide information and support. Some of these groups are run by patients or ex-patients themselves; others are organised by nurses or counsellors. They choose how often they meet, and their members may be available by telephone to support and encourage new patients. Sometimes even people who are not by nature great 'joiners', who usually avoid group activities, find that the opportunities for sharing their feelings – or just listening to other people's experiences – make them feel better. They feel that they can band together with others in a kind of joint enterprise to beat the disease.

Psychotherapy and hypnotherapy are professional services, and they should not be attempted by amateurs. They are useful for people who have serious psychological problems, and may well be suggested by a doctor as therapies which are useful in certain circumstances. For instance, some people who have had a bad experience with chemotherapy may begin to experience nausea as a conditioned response whenever they approach a hospital, or even when they watch a hospital programme on television. In that case, hypnotherapy can be used to change a distressing response, and help the patient escape from something which has gone beyond his or her conscious control.

Three useful mental techniques which you can practice yourself are relaxation, meditation and visualisation, though you may prefer to be taught these initially by an expert in a class or from a cassette tape. They can all have real and measurable effects on your pulse rate and blood pressure, and can be helpful to anyone suffering from stress, migraine, anxiety or certain digestive problems. They usually involve simple breathing exercises and concentration, letting thoughts and worries flow away from you and refusing to think about them, but keeping your attention on your breathing. Once you have mastered proper relaxation (it is not the same as just sitting or lying down and not moving much!) you can move on to the other techniques.

Meditation often involves deep relaxation, but moves into focusing the thoughts in certain directions. Those who have a religious faith usually focus on the person of God, Jesus or the Holy Spirit, or on the promises of God to care for his children. Others like to think about places where they have been very happy. Visualisation is a kind of extension of this: it involves the use of the imagination when you are deeply relaxed. Some therapists have encouraged cancer patients to imagine their bodies killing off the cancer cells; others encourage patients to visualise themselves getting stronger and healthier. Many people report good results from this, in terms of feeling fitter and happier.

Get physical

Another set of therapies which are generally acknowledged to be helpful are the physical ones which are mostly based around massage. Touch is important for everyone, whether it is a reassuring hand on the shoulder or a comforting hug. Massage has become increasingly popular in recent years, especially to relieve muscle pain and tension. Although it is probably most effective when performed by an expert, anyone can learn basic massage techniques. The only things to beware of are avoiding tender areas, and taking medical advice when using massage oils in cases where the skin may be sensitive after radiotherapy or chemotherapy.

Reflexology is a specialised form of foot massage, which has also been reported as reducing pain and tension; this must be performed by a trained therapist. Shiatsu is another form of massage, based on a Japanese tradition, which seems to be relaxing and energising.

Acupuncture is not based on conventional massage but similarly exerts pressure on certain points in the body, this time by inserting sterile needles into the skin. It is important that this is done by a trained therapist, since there have been cases of infection caused by poor hygiene during acupuncture. Although there is a whole philosophy of Chinese medicine underlying its theory, some Western doctors believe that they can understand some of its effects. During acupuncture the body releases natural chemicals which relieve pain and make the patient feel relaxed and well.

The theory of acupressure (pressure on particular points of the body) is also used to counteract nausea. Elasticated wrist bands with a small bead attached are used to apply light pressure to a point on the wrist, and are reported to be effective in treating nausea as a result of chemotherapy and even seasickness.

Medication

There are several kinds of treatment which amount to medication, taken by mouth in tablet or liquid form or applied to the skin. Homeopathy is another complementary therapy. Its practitioners do not claim to cure cancer but to alleviate symptoms and side-effects. Although the theory of homeopathy is not generally regarded as scientifically proven by doctors, many take the pragmatic view that it does no harm and it seems to have many beneficial effects, and a homeopathy service is available from some NHS hospitals and GPs.

Bach flower remedies are similar in that they use substances which are diluted many times – so many times that the original essences, extracted from flowers, are barely detectable. Many people believe that they help emotional and psychological symptoms; they are available from some chemists and health food shops.

Other herbal medicines should be regarded with greater caution. Many people labour under the delusion that anything which says 'herbal' or 'natural ingredients' on the label must be harmless: this is not so, any more than every 'artificial' substance is dangerous. For instance, one medication, derived from bitter almonds, claims to boost the immune system. In fact, when scientifically tested, it has been shown to release dangerously high levels of cyanide into the bloodstream. Some herbal medicines may be safe; others may interact with other medication you are taking. If you wish to try any of these therapies, you should always check with your GP or specialist first, and make sure that the therapist is properly qualified.

Diet

There is a developing body of evidence that the diet we eat has an effect, not only on our general health, but also on our risk of getting cancer. We mentioned in Chapter 1 some of the current advice about diet:

- eat plenty of plant-based foods (wholegrains and pulses)
- eat plenty of fruit and vegetables (preferably five servings a day)
- eat food which is low in saturated fat
- eat food which is low in salt
- avoid smoked, cured and charred foods.

This cannot guarantee that you will not get cancer, but you will be avoiding some of the known triggers.

However, some organisations have developed special diets which they suggest will help cancer patients. They are usually designed to get rid of toxins from the body, and they are often vegetarian (no meat, sometimes no fish) or vegan (no meat, fish or dairy products). A healthy diet will of course be helpful to you, but extreme or very limited diets should be treated with caution. A cancer patient who has lost a lot of weight or who has digestive trouble caused by other treatment may find such diets problematic. Cutting out all salt and sugar can make food very tasteless, at a time when you may need to be tempted to eat at all. Similarly, avoiding milk, cheese and eggs can remove useful sources of calories and protein just when your body needs building up. A sudden change to wholegrains and lots of fibre if you are not used to it can also put your digestion under stress.

Making healthy changes and improving your diet is probably a good idea, but such changes should be made gradually, and you should make sure that you are getting enough nutrition at all times. The dietician at the hospital will be able to help you. Diets which make wild claims for curing cancer on their own are unreliable. Two diets suggested to Roy required that the patient eat only grapes or only water melon for six months (I think he would have suffered from malnutrition as well as cancer by then).

Vitamins are another area where there is a lot of confusion. It is important that your diet delivers the right amount of vitamins to maintain health, and certain vitamins (beta-carotene, vitamin A, vitamin C and vitamin E) are thought to play a role in preventing cancer. As a result, some alternative therapists recommend megavitamin therapy. However, it is not necessarily true that because a small amount of something is good for you, therefore a large amount will be even better. In the case of most vitamin supplements which are available in tablet form, excess amounts are simply excreted by the body. Some of them, such as vitamins A and D, can be harmful if taken in large doses. One lady was told that cancer was caused by a lack of vitamin K, and instructed to drink a pint and a half of carrot juice every day. Apart from the risk of turning her skin orange, this would probably have made her very ill from an excess of vitamin D, had she followed it. In any case, there is as yet no evidence that those vitamins which are thought to protect the body against cancer are able to treat it once it has developed.

Beyond the fringe

You may be given other suggestions for helping yourself back to health. Like the various therapies listed above, they vary widely. Sometimes they are clearly sensible, like taking exercise which you enjoy, as often as you feel able. Doing anything you enjoy, whether it is listening to music, painting, walking or cycling, increases your feeling of well-being. Taking moderate exercise will stimulate your circulation and release the natural chemicals which make you feel relaxed and invigorated. As long as you don't exhaust yourself, this is good advice.

Other suggestions may be wilder. There may be some kind of rationale for winding copper wire around the legs of your bed, but I suspected that it wouldn't stand up to much scientific analysis. Many of these ideas depend more than a little on what you believe in. Indeed, there is a well-known effect called 'placebo', in which patients are given pills made of something harmless but ineffective (usually as part of a clinical trial to check the performance of another drug), and find that their symptoms have been relieved. The assumption is that the mind is very powerful: if you believe that something will make you feel better, it will probably do so. However, 'feeling better' is not the same as the cure of a serious illness, and the two should not be confused. Believing in the power of something may make your headache less worrying or your nausea recede; there is no evidence that it will shrink a tumour.

Other strange suggestions I have heard include fasting, enemas and colonic irrigation, tree hugging, sound therapy, and colour therapy (including drinking water which has been standing in a coloured glass). It is natural that you will be interested in anything which offers you a hope of improving your chances, but now, as much as ever before, you need to retain your hold on your common sense.

Belief in what?

If you look in the 'mind and spirit' section of any large bookshop nowadays, you will find a staggering range of ideologies, belief systems, religions and self-help systems on offer. Everything from *The Little Book of Calm* (keep calm, breathe deeply, don't get stressed, and your life will be better) to 'the healing power of crystals'. Now there is no doubt that science does not have the answer to everything, and that our minds have a power over our bodies. Nevertheless, if we allow ourselves to be swayed by every fashion that comes along, we live in a perpetual muddle. Extreme caution is advised!

Feng Shui suggests that putting a healthy plant in the 'wealth corner' of our house means that money will pour in. Believers in 'pyramid power' think that sitting in a pyramid structure will increase their energy. Millions of people read their 'stars' – predictions for everyday life made by astrologers – in daily newspapers and magazines each day, even though it is very unlikely that the same prediction will affect the millions of different lives which fall into each star sign. Yet others consult clairvoyants, mediums and psychics for guidance. As G.K. Chesterton said, when people stop believing in God, they don't then believe in nothing, they believe in anything – and everything. The Bible talks about people being 'tossed back and forth by the waves, and blown here and there by every wind of teaching.' (Ephesians 4:14)

Many books promise to make our lives wonderful overnight. They each claim to have a new formula for a happy life: follow its rules and you will become healthy, or successful, or calm, or wealthy, or whatever it is you think will make you happy. Unfortunately, there is a fatal flaw in the logic: health, success or money do not automatically guarantee happiness, as we see from the sad stories of rich and famous individuals who turn to drink or drugs to escape the emptiness of their lives.

Jesus, on the other hand, does not promise that anyone will be rich or successful; in fact, he deliberately chose some poor, uneducated working men to be his first followers. What he does promise, however, is that his followers are held securely in God's love. Anyone who is trying to follow his commandments is guaranteed a special kind of success: knowing that he or she is unique, created by God and loved by him for all time. God does not promise that we will be kept safe from illness or fear, but he does promise that we will not be overwhelmed by it. Certainly throughout Roy's illness we suffered all the ups and downs of treatment that went well and treatment that made him ill, hopes and fears and adjustments to a situation that was constantly changing. Yet through it all we knew that God was holding us in his hand, and that he would bring us through. Even in the worst times we had a kind of happiness deep within us, what Christians call joy, because we knew that even when death threatened it had no power over us.

Doing your own thing

Even if you have never had any interest in religion before, it may be something that interests you now. In the same way, you may never have taken any exercise, but find that it helps you to feel fitter and as though you are doing something constructive about getting well. People find all sorts of ways of helping themselves: one woman started an Open University course as a way of taking her mind off her illness and making her concentrate on something else.

Not everything that you choose to do will be focused on curing your cancer: some therapies are designed to make your symptoms milder, or just to improve your quality of life. No one knows how far the 'feel-good factor' can influence your health, but there is evidence that if you are reasonably optimistic, positive and relaxed you are giving your body the best, stress-free chance of getting on with fighting the cancer. At the same time you can suffer from too much pressure to be all of those things: constantly being told that you must 'think positive' and 'fight' can be wearing. You have to accept that you can't feel cheerful all the time, and there will be days when you feel less positive, but it isn't important.

Roy was a man who always saw the funny side of everything, and as a family we always laughed a lot, even through his illness. At the beginning of his chemotherapy he went upstairs to wash his hair, and then called us up to look: his hair had begun to fall out, and he had laid it out in clumps all along the side of the bath. 'Gives a whole new meaning to "Wash and Go",' he said. Later on, when he was baptised at our local church, he chose the hymn 'Be bold, be strong', which he said the congregation could sing as 'Be bald, be strong' in his case. Laughter is a great stress-buster, and always makes you feel better (again, scientific studies have shown that the beneficial physical effects are real). This does not mean that you have to embark on a new career as the family comedian, or try to cheer people up with an endless supply of jokes. However, remember that humour releases both tension and embarrassment, and that you can take problems seriously without being solemn about them.

You can help yourself by doing whatever suits you – whether it is laughing at a comedy video, praying, talking to your friends, or taking up a new hobby. You should, however, keep a sense of proportion. Always beware of anything that makes categorical claims about ensuring your survival, whether it is a medication, lifestyle or mental attitude. If there were a sure-fire cure available, everyone would know about it.

Part III

Looking Ahead

Look up with wonder.
Look back with gratitude.
Look around with love.
Look within with honesty.
Look ahead with anticipation.

Jim Graham

7. A Difficult Path

This book has been written to help cancer sufferers, and sets out to provide information about most of the things you may want to know about. In the case of incurable cancer, this may be something you don't want to know about! If that is the case, just don't read this chapter. If thinking about death will depress you, you don't have to do it. However, for those of us who have had to walk along this difficult path, it helps to have some sort of map of what we may meet along the way.

At the end of their treatment many people get a tentative 'all clear' from the doctors. I say tentative, because it is very hard for doctors to be sure that they have killed off or removed every last cancer cell, and as we know, any cancer cells left in the body will go on dividing, and the cancer will recur. Others will be told that there are definitely still some cancer cells present, but that they may lie dormant for years. The cancer check-ups for both groups will gradually get further and further apart, until (after five years or so) the doctors feel that they are no more likely to suffer a recurrence of the disease than anyone else is to develop cancer.

However, for some people there comes a time when the doctors tell them that their cancer has either spread or come back, and some of them may also be told that this time it is unlikely to be curable. These people suffer the same reactions as they did when diagnosed the first time, but with deeper levels of distress. They know what they are facing in terms of treatment, if that is what is offered, but they also face, once again, the fact that they may die.

Elvira Lowe suffered a recurrence of breast cancer five years after her first diagnosis and treatment. She says, 'I had a great sense of disappointment that the cancer had returned after five years, just when I thought it was all behind me. I was also saddened and upset that I had to have a mastectomy, and this was just as difficult to accept as the news that I had cancer. Now I find that living with the diagnosis of cancer is more difficult. I keep wondering if an unusual pain or symptom means that the cancer has recurred.' When Roy's cancer returned, we also felt disappointed. He had done so well, and championed the cause of other cancer sufferers; he felt as though he was letting them down.

Even when cancer is not curable, it may become like any other chronic illness: it is there in the background as a condition you have, but it is mostly not acute, and when it does become troublesome it can be controlled by a short burst of treatment. Certain cancers are so slow-growing that although they are undeniably present in your body, they are extremely unlikely to be the cause of your death, as you will almost certainly die of old age first!

It may seem ghoulish to talk like this about death and dying, but all of us will die one day. Cancer sufferers are merely being forced to face now what everyone has to face eventually: the fact of our mortality. Everyone's first question when they know they have cancer is, 'Am I going to die?' Whatever road their particular journey follows after that first diagnosis, they may eventually reach a point where they know that they are not going to recover.

Some people go on being willing to try anything and everything to cure or at least hold back their cancer. Others decide that there is a point where they want to stop, and they don't want to put their body through any more operations, tests or treatments. This is not necessarily a sign of 'giving up' on life; rather it may be a positive acceptance of what is happening, and an active choice to spend the time remaining in a way of your own choosing.

Even the amount of time remaining is almost impossible to predict. Many patients have been told that they are likely to live for another three months, and have gone on to live for two or three years, for most of which time they may be fairly well and active. Linda McCartney, who died of breast and liver cancer in 1998, was out riding her horse two days before her death. Many people have astounded their doctors by outliving all expectations, often in order to fulfil a personal ambition or to see through a family occasion such as Christmas or a wedding. It seems almost as though such people keep going by will power until the event is over, when they allow themselves to slip away peacefully.

Facing your fears

When you are walking along this difficult path of living with an incurable cancer, you may feel overwhelmed by the knowledge of your condition. The whole of society seems to work on the basis of investment in the future, whether it is buying insurance, planning for retirement, or even booking next year's holiday. You may feel that you have suddenly been excluded from normal life. Yet in spite of this, the reality is that everyone has to live one day at a time. The quality of today's experience is not really affected by how many tomorrows there may be.

I heard a lovely story of an elderly lady who went into her bank and was asked by a young cashier if she would like to take out life insurance. She replied, 'My dear, at my age I debate about buying a bunch of green bananas!'

The knowledge that your lifespan is limited forces you to face up to the fact of death. However, it may also bring to the surface a range of fears that are to do with the process of dying. A hundred years ago, people were more familiar with dying: when there were few hospitals, hospices or old people's and nursing homes, people were more likely to die at home among their family. Nowadays few of us have seen anyone who is near death, so we are that much more fearful of the unknown. When we have to face the prospect for ourselves, we may realise that we are afraid of what is involved in dying.

Pain

One fear may be that you will have to suffer great pain towards the end of your life, and the first thing to say is that this is certainly not inevitable. One in three cancer patients suffer no pain at all, and in the remaining cases, pain can be completely or mostly controlled in nine out of ten cases. Everyone's experience of pain is different, and so you should never be concerned about telling your doctor or nurse when you are in pain: there is no 'normal amount' of pain that you can be expected to experience, and you are certainly not being a nuisance or making a fuss if you tell them about your pain, or request a different dose of pain-killing medication.

The first aim of pain-killing drugs is to prevent pain, and they work better if you take them regularly, before the pain takes hold. If you wait for the pain to come back before you take them, you will suffer pain while you are waiting for the drug to be absorbed and start working. The dose should be enough to keep you pain-free until the next dose is due: if it does not, you should tell your doctor, so that you can be prescribed a higher or a more frequent dose, or a different drug.

You will not become addicted to your pain-killers. Relying on a drug for pain relief is not at all the same thing as addiction, and you will not become psychologically dependent on it. However, you should not stop taking your drugs suddenly: when you no longer need them, the doctor will gradually reduce your dose.

Pain relief is generally given by mouth, in the form of pills or syrup, but in emergencies it may be given by injection. For some patients it is more effective to deliver a continuous supply of a drug (usually morphine) into the body by using a syringe driver. This consists of a small pack which can be worn on a belt or kept by the bed, and a needle which delivers the drug painlessly under the skin or (occasionally) into a vein. The dose rate can be carefully measured and easily changed.

Living wills

One concern which often follows on from the use of painkillers in the case of terminal illness, is the use of very large amounts of such drugs and whether they shorten life. Euthanasia is mean the action of ending a person's life if they themselves request it; it is legal only in one state in Australia, and in Holland it is allowed in certain circumstances. It is not legal in the United Kingdom. There is ongoing public debate about 'assisted suicide' but currently this is still a criminal offence and all cases are investigated by the police. Many other countries have also rejected it: it is accepted that some people might like to choose when to end their lives, but such a system can too easily be abused by unscrupulous people, where issues such as inheritance or the cost of health care are involved.

In the UK what is accepted is something called the 'double effect': a doctor is permitted to deliver high levels of a drug – so high that the drug may be shortening the person's life – if the primary aim is the control of pain. This means that no one needs to fear suffering great pain at the end of their life, as the doctor is not prevented from delivering pain-relieving drugs.

It is also possible to arrange to make what is called a 'living will'. This document asks doctors to avoid making strenuous efforts to prolong your life if the eventual outcome is known to be terminal. For instance, if you know that you are dying from cancer, you may not wish to be resuscitated after a heart attack, or given treatment if you develop pneumonia. Many people make such wills to avoid unnecessary intervention is the last days or weeks of their life. Again, this is not the same as euthanasia, as you are not asking anyone to act to end your life, and it is your right to refuse treatment at any time.

Loss of activity

Another fear can be the loss of activity and independence. It is hard to face up to the fact that because of the cancer, or because of the side-effects of the treatment, you cannot do all the things you once took for granted. You may be unable to drive or even walk as far as you once did; you may become dependent on others to fetch your shopping or cook your meals. It can be difficult to accept these changes.

If you have very little energy, you may find that you have to establish priorities: arrange for visits to happen in the morning when you are fresh, and set aside time to rest in the afternoon. Make use of all the practical aids that are available from your occupational therapist: using a wheelchair may seem a drastic move, but it can give you independence and mobility when you need it; a hand-rail installed in the bathroom or a special toilet seat may enable you to go on caring for yourself.

If a time comes when you cannot manage intimate things like washing and toileting alone, you may find it easier to accept the more 'impersonal' help from a professional carer or nurse, for whom these actions are merely routine, than from your family or friends, who may find them embarrassing.

Being alone

Not everyone has family or friends who are willing or able to care for them, but you need not fear that you will be left alone. There is a whole range of services and individuals who are available to help out in cases of severe illness.

Your GP, as usual, is the first link in the chain. He or she has overall responsibility for prescribing your drugs and assessing your needs for medical and nursing care. The community or district nurses provide practical nursing services such as bathing and changing dressings. Other nurses include Macmillan nurses who make home visits, and Marie Curie nurses who may provide some day or night nursing. There are also home care teams who are based at hospitals, but who will make home visits.

Other support is available from occupational therapists and physiotherapists who work in the community as well as in hospitals, home helps who will do jobs in the home such as cleaning, shopping and cooking, and care attendants who will help with washing and dressing or just provide company. A social worker can visit to assess your needs and arrange for many of these services, and also sort out such things as adaptations to the home and special equipment, laundry and home care services and meals on wheels. They can also provide general advice, including financial information about benefits.

All these support services vary in their availability: some parts of the country are well served, but in others the level of provision is low. Enquire at your local Citizen's Advice Bureau or at your doctor's surgery to find out what is available where you live.

Staying at home

Many people, faced with the prospect of a terminal illness, wish to stay at home. If you are being discharged from hospital, you should do some advance planning, and try to arrange that as much support as you will need will already be in place. This may mean making contact with some of the people mentioned above, and sorting out what help you are likely to need. However, you should bear in mind that circumstances change, and that the level of support and help you require may increase or decrease according to how well you are feeling.

For instance, you may prefer to have a bed installed in a downstairs room, where you will feel more involved in the daily life of the household, but can retire to your room easily when you get tired. Other people may prefer to be upstairs and away from the noise and bustle of family life! Discuss frankly whether it is better for your partner to sleep in the same room or a separate one, and whether you will disturb each other.

If you are concerned about the people who will be caring for you, and worried that you will be putting too much strain on them, it may be a good idea to get them to talk to someone from Social Services separately. Most carers have a legal right to an assessment of their own needs when Social Services are deciding what help to offer you. See www.carers.org, the website of The Princess Royal Trust for Carers.

Hospice care

Your family, friends, social services and others may be able to meet all your needs, which is a fortunate situation. However, it may be the case that as your nursing needs increase, everyone, including yourself, is placed under increasing strain. If this is the case, then it may be time to consider whether hospice care would be appropriate for you, either as a short break from home, or for a longer period.

Hospices offer intensive care at the end of a patient's life, but they are not depressing places: if you think you might ever need their services, it is a good idea to arrange to visit one while you are still well enough to do so. Most hospices are friendly, comfortable places; they have a very high ratio of nurses to patients, and are quiet and restful. They often have many patients who are still active and mobile, and provide pleasant surroundings and activities for them, as well as home teams who will visit patients who spend most of their time at home, and use the hospice only for respite care. They are all free and accept patients of any faith and culture.

The main aims of hospice care are to relieve the symptoms and psychological stress of those approaching death, to help them to live as actively as possible in the meantime, and to support their families during the illness and afterwards when they are bereaved.

Dame Cicely Saunders, who founded St Christopher's Hospice in London in 1967, summarised the principle of hospice care like this:

> You matter because you are you.
> You matter to the last moment of your life,
> and we will do all we can
> not only to help you die peacefully,
> but to live until you die.

Most people who visit a hospice are encouraged by the cheering quality of love and care they experience there.

Practical considerations

At the very end of life few people are able to make complex decisions. In many cases the patient becomes gradually more deeply unconscious for a period of hours or days before death. It follows, then, that it is sensible to make some practical preparations while you are still able to do so.

The exact kind of preparation you need to make varies greatly, and depends on your personal situation. If you have a partner who will go on living in your home, you may need to think about which tasks were traditionally yours, and what he or she will have to take over. If you have always paid all the bills, does your partner know what needs paying and when? Do they know when the car needs servicing or how to contact the engineer to get the central heating fixed?

It is generally useful to make a list of important documents such as the title deeds of your house if you own it, your bank/building society account details, insurance and pension documents, tax and national insurance numbers, passport, driving licence, birth and marriage certificates and so on, and where to find them. You may want to list all the people who will need to be informed of your death, including old friends and also your employer, doctor and solicitor.

Some people like to make plans for their own funeral; it is a kindness to leave some instructions about whether you have strong feelings about burial or cremation, as families can agonise over doing 'the right thing', i.e. what you wanted. Sometimes talking about death in this way can help everyone to come to terms with what is happening.

One of the most important tasks is to make a will. If you have worked hard all your life for the things you have today, you will care about what happens to them in the future. Making a will ensures that you decide who receives your money and possessions; if you don't do this, the courts decide how to share out what you leave. Apart from the confusion and distress this can cause your family and loved ones, it may not reflect what you would have wanted at all.

A will is a legal document, and it has to be written down in the correct legal language. It is possible for you to write down what you want to happen, but if you use the wrong words the will could be declared invalid and your wishes ignored. It is always best to contact a solicitor for advice. It does not cost very much, but it is wise to ask around (from friends, family or the Citizen's Advice Bureau), and ask for an estimate of the costs before choosing a solicitor.

All you need to do is to list what you own (house, car, savings, cash, insurance policies and valuables). Think about what you owe, too, in terms of mortgages, credit cards, loans or hire purchase. Then work out whom you want to benefit from your will, including family and friends, and any charities. Take your lists to your solicitor, who will ensure that your wishes are written down and carried out.

None of these activities is morbid or necessarily depressing. In a way, you are ensuring your role in the future, no matter how far off that future may be. It can also be helpful to both you and your family if you can make preparations like this. It saves them worry and distress in the long term, and it may also help both them and you to have some peace of mind right now.

Thinking ahead

In his last illness Roy used to say, 'I'm not afraid of dying. Millions of people have done it, and I've never heard a complaint yet!' But we did talk about it, and think about it, and prepare for it. In many ways we felt that we were lucky, since we knew that he was going to die: we had time to share our feelings, and say things we wanted each other to know, apologise for the times things had gone wrong, and generally to make our peace with each other. So often in the busy rush of life, we don't make time to tell people how much we love them –

sometimes we are almost too embarrassed to do so. When someone is dying, all that gets swept away. We have the freedom to be open about our feelings that comes with an emotional crisis.

I am so very grateful that I had the privilege of that two and a half years with Roy after his cancer was first diagnosed. I was able to tell him how grateful I was that he had been such a good husband to me, and such a good father to our four children. I was able to tell him how much I loved him, and how sorry I was for all the foolish times in the early years of our marriage when we had argued over silly little things.

In the same way it can help to patch up any old quarrels and sort out any old grievances. If there are people you have lost touch with but would like to see, now is a good time to do it: a letter or phone call explaining about your illness can be the opening to a simple apology and a happier, more peaceful frame of mind. You may want to visit old friends or even places which hold special memories for you: now you can make the time, while you are still well enough to do things.

Some years ago Jill Dando, a young television presenter, was shot dead outside her house in the middle of an ordinary morning. The day after her death, a friend of mine looked casually at her watch, and then said, 'At this time yesterday, Jill Dando didn't know she had only one hour to live.' It seemed a ghoulish remark, but it made me think. If we knew we were about to die, what would we do? We wouldn't be worrying about whether we had been a success in life. We wouldn't be worrying about whether we had got all our work finished. We would be doing business with God and one another; with God, reaching out our hands to his fatherly love, and with our loved ones, making sure they knew how much we cared for them.

Knowing you have a terminal illness is in many ways an unbearable grief. But we do bear it, and come to recognise that knowing we are going to die is also a privilege. We have the opportunity to make our wrong relationships right, to sort out any unfinished business, and to ensure that we can leave this world with a clean heart and as few regrets as possible. There may be old wounds to heal, and harsh words to repent. We can also make things easier for those we leave behind. We may need to reassure them that we forgive them for anything they may have done in the past, which would otherwise cause them pain when we have gone.

Although we have no knowledge of what lies on the other side of death for us, Christians believe that they are going home to their Father, who loves them. They believe that they will finally see Jesus, the Lord they serve here on earth. Other faiths have other ideas, and many people simply believe that death is the end of their existence. However, we all have some idea what faces our loved ones when we have died: for them life will go on, but without us. For some people this thought is unbearably sad. Others want to make some preparation to help their families and friends, perhaps by writing letters or making video recordings. One young mother made scrapbooks for her children, containing little mementoes of their babyhood – snips of hair from their first haircut and so on – together with lots of photographs of each of them with her, so they would always remember how much she had loved them.

Valuing you

A cancer nurse once told Roy, 'If anyone ever tells you there's nothing more that can be done, don't believe them. There's always something we can do to make you feel better. It may not be a cure, but we can give you pain relief and control your symptoms, and put you back in charge of your own life.'

This is one area where the hospice movement has helped to refocus attitudes to patient care. A dying patient is no longer one for whom medicine has failed, but rather an individual at a particular stage in life's journey. The hospice affirms life, and recognises dying as a normal process. Because of this, the hospice offers 'skilled companionship' at this stage, recognising the unique importance of each individual, promising to stay alongside each one until they die, and encouraging them to see that their life still has meaning and direction.

The plain fact is that ultimately everyone dies. Making an effort to feel better today – whether that means alleviating some symptom, or being absorbed in writing an important letter, or just enjoying the sunshine – is worthwhile. Even if those things do not change the outcome, that does not mean that the effort was a failure, or not worth making. Each day of your life is important. However limited your powers may become, even if you are confined to bed and unable to do much for yourself, you are able to go on living and loving until the end.

One man, who had had part of his lung removed, told me, 'I made a decision when I came round from the operation: I'm going to get on with this. I may be going to die in the end, but I'm going to die living, not live dying.'

8. Getting Clear of Cancer

Cancer no longer means death. Cancer treatments are getting better and better, and more and more people are surviving. Around 50% of all cancer sufferers do not die within five years, and for many common cancers the survival rates are much higher (95% for testicular cancer). Research by Macmillan Cancer Support ('Living after Cancer: median cancer survival time', November 2011) found that many cancer patients survive their disease nearly six times longer than they did 40 years ago. This is good news. Yet when many cancer patients are discharged from the hospital, they are left with a curious uncertainty: no one has told them they are cured.

This is partly because, as we have seen, it is extremely difficult to be sure that every last cancer cell has been eradicated from the body, and any remaining cancer cells may start dividing again at any time. Doctors cannot guarantee that this will not happen. Instead, they have a variety of terms for describing the situation after treatment is completed. 'Partial remission' means that a tumour has shrunk to less than half its original size, and has stayed that way for a month or more. 'Complete remission' means that a tumour has been removed by surgery, or appears to have disappeared completely after radiotherapy or chemotherapy, and that all tests which were previously abnormal are now clear. After that, they begin to talk about 'disease-free survival' – how long a patient survives with no sign of any tumour.

Different cancers tend to recur after different time periods: certain cancers almost always recur (if they are going to do so) during the first five years, so if you remain disease-free for longer than that, your cancer is less likely to come back. Other cancers, however, have a pattern of recurrence over a much longer period, so you may be encouraged to have check-ups at monthly intervals, then six-monthly, then yearly intervals for ten or fifteen years.

Mary Blackmore says,

> After I completed treatment for breast cancer (including surgery, chemotherapy and radiotherapy) several people asked what would happen next. 'What's the prognosis?' 'How long have you got?' 'Are you clear or is it likely to come back?' I didn't know what to say.
>
> When I asked the oncologist about this he had a quite definite reply. 'Just tell them we don't know. But next time, it's just as likely to be one of them as it is you.' In other words – I am no more likely to get cancer again than anyone else who has never had it. He told me that if I noticed any new symptom that lasted more than three weeks I should contact his department at once. 'Otherwise,' he said, 'I'll see you in two years' time!' That gave me the confidence to get on with life, and be thankful for every new day.

One patient with lung cancer was told after five years that all his tests were clear. He did not need any more check-ups, but he was advised to return annually anyway. 'I got really worried then,' he says. 'I thought there was something they weren't telling me.' In fact, this was simply prudent advice designed to set his own mind at rest, not to cause him extra worry.

Out on your own

When a course of treatment has been completed and you are discharged from hospital, you may feel unexpectedly low. You may be anxious to put the whole episode behind you and think of your cancer as 'over', but as we have seen above, doctors are extremely unwilling to use the word 'cured'. You may be keen to get back to normal, but after such an experience and in such conditions, life is not really normal.

Going home from hospital presents you with yet another set of adjustments. In hospital you have to make very few decisions for yourself; there are doctors and nurses and other staff to rely on. You may have become somewhat 'institutionalised', and it is something of a shock to have to think about what you are going to cook for dinner, and make sure that you have the energy to prepare a meal. You may still be feeling ill and tired from the effects of the treatment. Above all, the fact of your cancer may still be uppermost in your mind, and it may be difficult to be cheerful and ordinary, and not to keep talking about it. Yet that is just what your family and friends may be longing for. They want the whole episode to be over, but it is hard for you to take up all your old roles immediately.

Regular visits to the hospital, although intruding on your time and energy, have nevertheless provided a structure to your life as a cancer patient. During your treatment you have had the security of the whole hospital system and the support of experts. Now, on your own outside the hospital, you may feel nervous and insecure.

One patient said, 'I was given the 'all clear' from lung cancer after ten years, and told I didn't have to come to hospital any more. It was the first day of the rest of my life. In fact, it was just about the most worrying day of my life. I didn't have any support any more. Now no one was checking up on me. How would I know if I was getting ill again?'

Even after you have been discharged, you may still go on being afraid that your cancer will return. You may wake at night worrying: every minor illness seems like the start of another tumour. The answer is to write down all your worries, and the next day, ring your cancer nurse or even the ward where you were treated. Help and advice is available, if you seek it out.

On the other hand, once the initial period of check-ups is over, you might find that you don't want to think about it any more. Asking for extra check-ups from your GP might worry you and make you keep thinking about your cancer unnecessarily. If that's the case, just ignore it, and go back to the doctor only if you have some symptom which needs investigation.

Money matters

There are other complications involved in getting back to normal after a serious illness. You may have financial difficulties.

Betty Napper, says, 'When I was being treated for ovarian cancer my husband Jack came to visit me in hospital a lot, but he didn't get paid for the time he took off work. By the time I came out of hospital we were really hard up. We took in lodgers to help with the money, though I don't know how I did it – I was still having chemotherapy, and I didn't feel too good a lot of the time. Jack used to get up early and help me with the breakfasts before he went to work. We got ourselves straight in the end.'

Financial problems cannot be ignored, as debts have a way of increasing. Betty was able to solve her temporary financial crisis herself, but you may not be well enough or find the opportunities to do this. Fortunately, help is available. If you have trouble paying your bills, rent or community charge, you should contact a social worker or the Citizen's Advice Bureau for money advice. This is entirely confidential, but may help you to sort things out. If you find it hard to pay your mortgage, you should contact the manager of the bank or building society at once. Both organisations will sometimes suspend payments for a few months or arrange for you to pay at a lower rate for a time, until you get sorted out, especially if you have a letter from a social worker explaining the circumstances.

There are some charities which can help with the loan or purchase of special equipment if you need it. These include Macmillan Cancer Relief, the Red Cross and the Independent Living Fund.

The Citizen's Advice Bureau or a social worker can also tell you whether you are entitled to state benefits, how much you may get and how to apply. The rules are complex and change frequently, so it is a good idea to get individual advice. Don't rely on the leaflets you can pick up in the doctor's surgery or post office: there are lots of obscure corners to the benefits system! You may be able to work part-time and still qualify for benefits, but you need to know exactly what your situation is, in order to do this without breaking the law. The government has a telephone advice service called the Benefit Enquiry Line which gives confidential information to enquirers.

Insurance is another area where you may find unexpected difficulties. If you already have life insurance, your company may not be willing to increase the value of your policy for some time. You may also find it impossible to take out new life insurance for two or three years after your illness, and when you do, the premiums are likely to be high. This is because insurance companies like to keep their own risks to a minimum, and once you have had cancer, for the first five years or so you are at a greater risk than other people of being ill again. An independent financial adviser should be able to contact a wide range of companies for you and find you the best deal. The British Insurance Brokers Association should be able to find someone to help you with travel insurance and mortgages.

Back to work

If your cancer is diagnosed while you are working, your rights are protected by law. Depending on your contract of employment, your employer probably has to hold your job open for you during your treatment. You don't have to tell your employer that you are having tests for cancer, but it is obviously better to tell the full facts as soon as you know them. Then you can find out what benefits you are entitled to, what medical certificates you need, and how long you can be off work on full or part pay. You can also expect your employer to make reasonable arrangements to help you if you wish to carry on working.

If you should be sacked on health grounds, you can challenge your dismissal as unfair under certain circumstances, depending on how long you have been working in that job.

Everyone is different in their reaction to illness and treatment, and so you have to trust your own feelings about when you are ready to go back to work. Make sure that your energy level and stamina are up to a full day's work, if that is what is required: one man reported that he took on a job that was more than he could manage, and he had to give it up. That was a real blow to his self-esteem, and it was a long while before he dared try again, as he was afraid of letting people down. Betty Napper went back to her part-time job as soon as she could: 'I used to feel very sick the first day after the chemotherapy, so my employer said that I needn't come in to work on the weeks I had treatment. I worked all the rest of the time, though.' Some people see returning to work as a mark of returning to 'ordinary' life; others find that their priorities have changed, and that they are no longer prepared to give so much of their time and energy to their career – they may want to change to a lower-key job.

You may be looking for work because you lost your job or decided to resign during your illness. Whatever your reasons, applying for a new job raises some more awkward questions. You do not need to tell anyone the details of your illness, but if there are questions about your health on the application form, or if someone asks you about your health in an interview, you should be truthful. If you conceal important information, you could later be dismissed. If you have prepared a curriculum vitae, or if you are asked about your employment history, a potential employer will see that there is a gap in your work record.

It's a good idea to be ready with your answers in advance. At any job interview you have to sell yourself and your ability to the job: you need to emphasise your past experience and your general good health now, and make it clear that your doctors consider your treatment to have been a success.

Changing perspectives

The people who make the best recoveries from cancer are often those who find ways of getting on with life – working when possible, doing as many normal tasks as they can, even planning for the future and planting bulbs for the spring (or a tree!). They are not blocking out the fact of their cancer but living with it, 'putting it on the back burner' while they get on with life. They know that they have had cancer, and they know that there is a chance that it will recur, but in the meantime they concentrate on each day as it comes, and think about their cancer only occasionally.

They also go on getting fun out of life. One man told his support group meeting, 'Someone told me it was good to have a tot of whiskey before going to bed. I tried it and it did me good. In fact, it does me so much good, now I go to bed six times a day!'   I have visited a lot of support groups, and I'm always amazed at the amount of laughter that goes on. Time after time people tell me that having cancer has changed all their perspectives on life. They are less worried about what other people think, and they measure 'success' differently. 'The important things in life aren't "things" at all', as one woman said.

They also tend to be more easy-going: when you have experienced serious illness, you measure trivial irritations on a different scale. On a scale of one to ten, with dying at the top, the dog walking mud over your clean floor doesn't even rate half a point – not worth shouting at him.

It is said that happiness is the gap between what you expect and what you get. If you expect a day to be dull and it turns out much better – the sun shines, you go out for a good meal or you meet an old friend – then you feel extra happy. When you have been confined to bed in a hospital ward, being fit enough for a walk round the garden can give you great pleasure. Once you have had a brush with illness and death, everything looks better than you expected. Roy said that he never minded standing waiting for a train in the rain: 'At least I'm alive to stand here and get wet!'

I think this is why cancer patients love life. They notice things in a new way, they are aware of the beauty of the world around them and the love of their families and friends, and they live life more intensely than ever before. This is not meant to be a sentimental 'there's always a silver lining' sort of philosophy. Angela Wilkie (who wrote *Having Cancer and How to Live with It*, Hodder & Stoughton) said that she was fed up with reading books which told her how cancer could lead to a fuller understanding of life, or spiritual growth, or true freedom, and she got angry at being 'told how to react'. (Roy would have identified with that!) Yet when she had expressed her anger and pain at having cancer, she clearly found herself with a new appreciation of the preciousness of life, and also a great compassion for others who were suffering the same fears and difficulties she went through.

Some people who have had cancer get irritated at being told, 'Just live one day at a time. Any one of us could die tomorrow.' They reply that there is a world of difference between a fit person's expectation of life (even being run over by a bus isn't all that likely!) and that of someone with cancer. Yet how they interpret 'living one day at a time' varies widely. For some people, it means being constantly aware of death, and they resent the fact that they have lost, perhaps for ever, the healthy person's ability to regard the possibility of death as remote. They allow it to affect everything they do. Other people take 'living one day at a time' to mean making the most of every day, and living life to the full. These are the people who are able to say, as I heard one woman say, 'Cancer is a spiritual gift.' She was in no way a religious person, but she felt that she was much more aware than ever before of the richness of the precious gift of life.

Making sense of it

So how do we make sense of this overwhelming experience that we have been through? Does it affect our everyday lives, or do we simply recover, and go back to living our lives in exactly the same way as before? The comments above suggest that few people do that. Most people who have been through the experience of having cancer and getting clear of it, find that their changed perspectives suggest something different.

Most of us feel we need some sense of direction, a belief that whatever life brings, we are held securely by some sense of purpose. It was this belief that kept us going throughout Roy's illness. We believed that 'nothing can separate us from the love of God', and that our lives do indeed have a purpose. That purpose is summed up in the teaching of Jesus: he cleverly reduced the long list of ten commandments which are given in the Old Testament, to two simple ones which are their essence: that we should love God with all our hearts, and that we should love our fellow human beings. For Roy, at the end of his life, that meant that he had to do all he could to help other cancer sufferers.

He had found that the publicity which surrounded his own illness made others feel better – sometimes just by making it an acceptable topic of conversation, and bringing it out of the realms of something embarrassing into ordinary life. He also knew that as a celebrity, he was able to attract publicity for a good cause. The result was the Cause for Hope appeal for research into lung cancer, which raised £1.2 million on his 'Tour of Hope'.

On 29 March 1996 I laid the foundation stone of the building that was to become the Roy Castle International Centre for Lung Cancer research in Liverpool. A wonderfully light, airy, pleasant building to work in, it is dedicated to the study and eventual elimination of lung cancer. It is a wonderful memorial to the joyful dedication of his life to making things better for all the others coming after him, who may be able to benefit from the work that goes on there.

Other cancer patients have felt similarly driven to do something to make a difference for other people with the same illness. Heather Mann says,

> In July 2003 I was treated for colon cancer ... two years later the doctors found a small lesion on my liver. During the subsequent operation and a further gruelling course of chemotherapy I valued the caring support and professionalism of the medical staff of the Royal Marsden Hospital. Their attitude was always reassuring and positive. Yet as a Christian, the sustaining power, strength and peace of my Heavenly Father was my main support, and the prayers and love of my family, church and friends helped me enormously.

> When I next saw my consultant, he pointed out that there was no local support group for liver cancer. With the help of Macmillan Cancer Support I set up a group called 'Livagain' – the name serves to emphasise that the liver regenerates after damage, and that in spite of such a traumatic experience, hope and new life can be regained. Nine years on, I am a living testimony!

As I travel around the country visiting support groups, patient networks and charity shops, I am continually struck by the fact that all these organisations are staffed by people who have experienced cancer in some way – either directly or through family or friends. So many people seem to demonstrate this same urge to make a difference, to make things better for other people, and to pass on whatever comfort and care they themselves have received from others.

It seems as though this is one way in which people make sense of the experience of cancer for themselves. They do not want to feel that their pain and distress were just meaningless, a random set of events in one person's life. Rather they want to feel that something useful has come out of it all; that they can share their experiences with others, or help support the doctors and nurses who supported them when they needed it.

Perhaps this is why all these places are always so full of fun, laughter, and loving concern.

Where do we go from here?

You may be one of the people for whom getting clear of cancer means doing something extraordinary that you would never otherwise have done: perhaps for yourself, like climbing a mountain, going on a cruise, or taking up painting, or for other people, like fund-raising for charity. Or you may be someone who is longing just for life to be really dull again – and how we appreciate ordinariness unpunctuated by hospital visits. Whichever you are, you can be sure that life will never be quite the same again.

You have seen how precious life and your loved ones appear when you think you might lose them. And you have been forced to confront the big questions of life – why are we here? What is valuable in life? What happens when we die?

When we have faced cancer, we have also faced the ultimate challenge of life – death. One reason why so many people refuse to think about cancer, or make it a taboo word, or avoid us in the street, is that they are afraid of being brought close to that reality. However, I believe that if we trust in a loving God we do not need to fear. We know that we and those we love are held safe in God's hands, and that nothing can separate us from His fatherly love (Romans 8:39).

Roy eventually died of cancer, but he was not defeated by it. He was not afraid of dying, and so he lived life to the full, trusting that when his time came, God would take him home. His last years were full of joy, thankfulness, fun and useful work, helping other people. All of us, healthy or ill, can do no more than that. I aim to live my life in a similar way, and I pray that you may, too.

9. Into the Future

Cancer patients have two urgent questions to ask: Will there ever be a cure for cancer? and Will it come soon enough to help me? The answer to both of them depends largely on the researchers.

The history of disease control is the history of medical research: as we have learned to understand the causes of illness and the mechanisms by which illness develops in the body, so we have been able to discover methods of curing it. It was the understanding of bacteria and the way they grow and multiply which led to the discovery of the antibiotics which can destroy them. A hundred years ago, smallpox and diphtheria were dreaded diseases; now, thanks to vaccines and drug therapies, they have both been virtually eliminated. There is no reason why we should not conquer cancer in the same way.

Prevention

We have already discovered some of the causes of many kinds of cancer, which have been mentioned earlier in this book. Forty years ago, no one thought there were any health risks associated with smoking tobacco: indeed, some of the very early advertisements suggested that it could be beneficial! Nowadays, no one needs to be in any doubt that smoking accounts for at least 90% of lung cancers, and is a contributory cause of many other cancers. Thirty years ago, sunburn was thought to be nothing more than a passing inconvenience: now it is known that sun damage to the skin can cause skin cancer.

Medical research has taught us these facts and many more about the causes of cancer, and as a result, there is a chance that we may be able to prevent many cancers in the future. If there are factors which increase the likelihood of people developing cancer, then by discovering more about them, and by making sure that people know about them, we may be able to protect people better in the future.

It has to be said, though, that it is not easy to persuade people of such risks: in spite of all the knowledge about the dangers of sun damage, many people still lie on the beach in the hottest part of the day, using only a tiny amount of sunscreen, because they think that having a suntan makes them look good. Similarly, it is difficult to persuade people not to start smoking (most people begin smoking as children: very few adults start smoking). And because of the addictive properties of nicotine, it is very hard for them to give up once they have started. So as well as research into the causes of cancer, we need to find out what are the most effective ways of getting the warnings across. We need to discover how we can help people to understand risk and how to protect themselves, and then produce effective publicity campaigns to get the message heard.

Preventing cancer requires research, development, staff and publicity: and it all costs money.

Detection

But what about the people who already have cancer, but do not know it? Most patients have the best chance of cure if their cancer is discovered at an early stage, especially before it has begun to spread to other parts of the body. There is a much better chance of getting rid of one localised tumour than of managing to kill off every last cancer cell in two or three locations. Early detection of cancer could save many lives.

Once again, research is required. many organisations are working hard on this problem, in respect of many different cancers. As we said earlier, cancer is not really a single disease but about 200 different ones, which all develop and spread in a similar way. So the symptoms of colon cancer are quite different from the symptoms of leukaemia, and in any case, many patients have no noticeable symptoms at all until their cancer is quite advanced. There is not yet a single simple method of detecting cancer, yet this would be invaluable.

However, great strides forward are being made. Gene research is a promising avenue, and genetic counselling is available for people with a strong family history of certain cancers.

Towards a cure?

We may be able to prevent many cancers in the future, and detect quickly those we cannot prevent, but what then? Is there any hope of a cure?

What is needed is a profound understanding of the behaviour of cells when they begin their strange alteration from healthy normal cells into cancerous ones. Then we may have some hope of preventing, retarding or reversing the changes. Scientists have discovered some of the key steps that turn healthy human cells into tumours: if they can build on these findings, they may be able to develop drugs which will block the growth of tumours. This is encouraging, but such findings emerge from research programmes lasting ten, fifteen or twenty years. You can see how long all these projects take: cancer researchers cannot afford to be in a hurry! However, that is just the opposite of cancer patients: they cannot afford to wait.

This kind of research offers real hope that we will conquer cancer one day in the near future – how near, depends very much on how much funding is available. There are many charities working at the forefront of cancer research, not in competition but in collaboration, trying to extend our knowledge of how cancer works and how it can best be treated.

Patient support

There are other concerns, too. What happens to all those cancer patients while they are waiting so eagerly for the researchers to do their work and come up with the cure? They need to know what is happening to their bodies, how to cope with their symptoms, and how to live with their fears. This book is a small contribution to the fund of information they need. Many of the cancer charities also provide information – sometimes about cancer in general, sometimes in-depth information about specific cancers and their related problems. They produce books, booklets, leaflets, posters, telephone helplines, internet websites – all sorts of ways of explaining about cancer, its causes and its treatment.

Many of them provide nursing care in and out of hospital, delivered by nurses who often care for and support the whole family as they face a difficult time together. They provide hospices and day-care centres where patients can be treated, cared for, and even pampered with beauty treatments and massages. They run patient support groups where patients can meet together and share their experiences and realise that they are not alone; often these are staffed by nurses or other specialist helpers. They also work to educate the public about cancer prevention and detection, and healthcare professionals about the latest developments in cancer care.

What's it worth?

The cost of all this activity is colossal, and almost all of it is funded by voluntary donations. (A few charities work in collaboration with the NHS when they are providing nursing care.) The cancer charities are doing wonderful work on every front, and yet they often have to make difficult decisions because of lack of money. They cannot provide nursing help to everyone who would like support to enable them to stay in their own home, if there is not enough money to pay the nurses. They cannot explore new avenues for cancer research if there is not sufficient funding to buy equipment or pay scientists. They are providing real help on a daily basis to thousands of patients, and real hope for a cure in the future.

Roy spent the last months of his life promoting cancer research. He knew that the work would be too late to help him, but he knew that it could help others in the future. No one would have blamed him if he had said, 'Sorry, but I'm very ill. Someone else can help now.' Instead he worked on tirelessly, using the fame he had built up over the years for a real and serious purpose: to raise funds to work for a cure. As he said in an interview: 'I can't give up now. There are 40,000 other lung cancer patients all pulling on the rope with me, and I can't let them down.'

Research is vitally important if we are ever to find a cure – for cancer in general and the many different types of the disease. Anyone who has either survived cancer or who has a loved one who has been treated for it will be passionate about raising funds to support research. If one in three of us will be diagnosed with cancer at some point, almost everyone will be affected by it; we need to keep fundraising so that future generations will not fear cancer as those in the past have done.

I don't ask for donations to any specific charity. Every one of the cancer charities is doing wonderful work. Any one of them would be grateful for whatever you can spare: your money, your time, your energy or your enthusiasm to help the cause forward. There are dozens of ways of giving: by covenant (which reclaims some money from the tax man), by payroll giving (where your employer does the work of passing on money from your salary), by legacy in a will, by banker's order, by cheque, by cash donation into a collecting box, or by volunteering your help at a charity shop or collecting day.

Your help can be part of this great effort in which we are all involved: to bring hope for the future, for all of us.

Useful Addresses

Action Cancer

www.actioncancer.org

Action Cancer is based in Northern Ireland and is a local organisation dedicated to cancer research, patient support and early detection. It has a special programme for the detection of breast cancer, including a mobile clinic, and also runs a men's health clinic.

Benefits Agency Helpline

www.directgov.uk

Helpline: 0911 775 0159

This is a free enquiry line for people on benefits and their carers. The line is open on weekdays during office hours.

Breast Cancer Care

www.breastcancercare.org.uk

Helpline: 0808 800 6000

Breast Cancer Care provides a national helpline; talks, courses, local support, telephone support online discussions and an aftercare service. It aims to offer information and support to patients, their families and friends, the public, healthcare professionals and the media.

British Homoeopathic Association

www.britishhomeopathic.org

The BHA provides information on homoeopathy and encourages further development of this natural system of medicine. It provides downloadable fact sheets and articles and information on how to get treatment.

British Insurance Brokers Association

www.biba.org.uk

BIIBA is the trade association for the insurance broking sector. Their members are registered and regulated under an Act of Parliament.

British Red Cross Society

www.redcross.org.uk

The British Red Cross doesn't just help out in major emergencies: it also supports people on their discharge from hospital, and loans medical equipment on a short-term basis.

Cancer Black Care

www.cancerblackcare.org.uk

Tel: 020 8961 4151

Cancer Black Care Information Centre offers comprehensive support service to all members of the community, who are affected by cancer. It offers a safe confidential, neutral place, where service users, carers and families and friends can meet to support each others' cultural and emotional needs.

CancerHelp UK

www.cancerhelp.cancerresearchuk.org

Helpline: 0808 800 4040

CancerHelp UK is the patient information website of Cancer Research UK. It provides a free information service about cancer and cancer care for people with cancer and their families.

Cancer Research UK

www.cancerresearchuk.org

Helpline: 0808 800 4040

Cancer Research UK conducts research into all aspects of cancer, and is delivering results that are already saving lives. It aims to further the understanding of the biology and causes of cancer, to develop new approaches for preventing and treating cancer, and to improve the quality of life for cancer patients.A cancer information nurse team is available to answer questions in confidence (please note the team are unable to make a diagnosis or offer a medical opinion).

CCLASP

www.cclasp.net

Tel: 0131 467 7420

Children with Cancer and Leukaemia, Advice and Support for Parents (CCLASP) is an Edinburgh based children's charity. CCLASP helps children and teenagers who have cancer or leukaemia. CCLASP also helps diagnosed families express and share with each other the feelings and anxieties of having a child with a life threatening illness.

CLAN Cancer Support

www.clanhouse.org

Helpline: 0330 440 2526

Cancer Link Aberdeen & North (CLAN) is an independent charity for anyone affected by any type of cancer at any time from diagnosis onwards. Based at CLAN House in Aberdeen, it covers the whole of Grampian, Orkney and Shetland.

Colostomy Association

www.colostomyassociation.org.uk

Helpline   0800 3284257

BCA represents the interests of people with a colostomy: it provides support, reassurance and practical information to anyone who is about to have, or already has a colostomy. A telephone and letter helpline are available, together with a directory of support groups, products and services.

Carers UK

www.carersuk.org

Helpline: 0808 808 7777

CarersUK is the voice of carers: it raises awareness at all levels of government and society of the needs of carers; provides carers with information and advice; offers a wide range of information on all aspects of caring; and supports carers with a network of branches and groups throughout the UK.

Cruse Bereavement Care

www.crusebereavementcare.org.uk

Helpline: 0844 477 9400

Cruse helps anyone who has been bereaved by providing 'someone to talk to'; groups where bereaved people can meet and talk; information on practical, financial and emotional aspects of bereavement; training, support and information for volunteers. It has a nationwide network of local groups.

DIAL UK

www.dialuk.info

Tel: 01302 310123

DIAL UK is the national organisation for a network of around 120 local Disability Information and Advice Line services run by and for disabled people. Last year DIALs helped over a quarter of a million disabled people. DIAL information and advice services are based througout the UK and provide information and advice on all aspects of living with a disability, including welfare benefits, community care, equipment, independent living, mobility and transport, discrimination, holidays and much more.

Disabled Living Foundation

www.dlf.org.uk

Helpline: 0845 130 9177

DLF is a national charity that provides impartial advice, information and training on daily living aids. It offers information and advice on disability equipment; it runs a database of information and provides an equipment directory and a range of publications. Staff answer personal enquiries, and demonstrate equipment at the London Demonstration Centre.

Everyman

http://everyman-campaign.org

Everyman's mission is to stamp out prostate and testicular cancer. They try to achieve this by helping everyone to recognise the tell-tale signs and understand the importance of treatment. In increasing this awareness they also hope to raise money to fund their life-saving research.

Evangelical Alliance

eauk.org

Tel: 020 7207 2100

The Evangelical Alliance is a wide-ranging group of churches of many denominations. If you would like help in finding a church to visit or attend, or just a Christian to talk to, ring the number given above.

Hospice Information Service

www.helpthehospices.org.uk

Tel: 020 7520 8222

The Hospice Information Service provides an enquiry service, information about hospice care, a searchable directory of hospices and palliative care services and a weekly e-newsletter.

Independent Living Fund

www.dwp.gov.uk/ilf

Tel: 0845 601 8815

The ILF93 Fund is a trust set up and financed by central government. Its aim is to support long-term independent living for disabled people by helping them live at home instead of in residential care.

Institute for Complementary and Natural Medicine

www.i-c-m.org.uk

ICNM provides the public with information on all aspects of the safe and best practice of complementary medicine through its practitioners, courses and research. It administers the British Register of Complementary Practitioners.

Institute of Family Therapy

www.ift.org.uk

Tel: 020 7391 9150

The Institute supports and helps families or couples who are experiencing difficulties, including illness and caring.

Leukaemia Care

www.leukaemiacare.org.uk

Helpline: 08088 010 444

Leukaemia CARE exists to provide vital care and support to all those whose lives have been affected by leukaemia, lymphoma, myeloma and the allied blood disorders. Their work includes the welfare of families and carers, as well as that of patients.

Look Good, Feel Better

www.lookgoodfeelbetter.co.uk

Tel: 01372 747500

Look Good, Feel Better is a national support programme offering skincare and make-up workshops and self-help materials for women to help combat the visible side effects of cancer treatment and, in turn, boost self-esteem and wellbeing.

Lymphoedema Support Network

www.lymphoedema.org

Helpline: 020 7351 4480

The Lymphoedema Network provides support and information; works towards the availability of better resources for treatment; maintains contact with healthcare professionals and promotes a network of support groups throughout the UK. It offers a telephone helpline, regular newsletters, up-to-date information and a range of publications.

Lymphoma Association

www.lymphomas.org.uk

Helpline: 0808 808 5555

The Association provides support and information on a range of issues to anyone with lymphatic cancer and their families, carers and friends. It organises a national network of patient support groups.

Macmillan Cancer Support

www.macmillan.org.uk

Helpline: 0808 808 0000

Macmillan Cancer Support helps people who are living with cancer. By working closely with people with cancer, their families and communities, they aim to develop services which reflect people's real needs and wishes. They also share their expertise with a wide range of health and social care providers, leading by example and inspiring others to meet their standards.

Although best known for their nurses, their increasing range of services includes specialist health and social care professionals; information and support services; grants and money advice; carer support services; self-help and support services; campaigning; and education, development and support services.

Maggie's

www.maggiescentres.org

Tel: 0131 537 3131

Maggie's Centres are a network of drop-in centres across the UK for anybody who has, or who has had cancer. They are also for their families, their friends and their carers. The aim of Maggie's Centres is to help people with cancer to be as healthy in mind and body as possible and enable them to make their own contribution to their medical treatment and recovery. They allow people to address all aspects of living with cancer. They can share their experiences with others in similar situations and, with professional help, inform themselves about the medical realities of their disease.

The friendly environment of the centres, close in each case to a major cancer hospital treatment centre, invites people to take time out and gives them a non-institutional place they can call their own.

Marie Curie Cancer Care

www.mariecurie.org.uk

Tel: 0800 716146

Marie Curie is a comprehensive cancer care charity, providing nursing care and support; medical, nursing and day centres; research to investigate the causes, prevention and early detection of cancer; and education for the public and healthcare professionals, all free of charge.

New Approaches to Cancer

www.anac.org.uk

Helpline: 0800 389 2662

New Approaches to Cancer aims to promote the benefits of holistic and self-help methods of healing for cancer patients. A referral system and information service operate, directing people with cancer to their nearest sources of help.

Orchid

www.orchid-cancer.org.uk

Helpline: 0203 465 6105:

Orchid exists to save men's lives from testicular, prostate and penile cancers, through pioneering research and promoting awareness. The charity is dedicated to funding research into, and awareness about, the cancers that uniquely affect men – their prevention, diagnosis and treatment. It has produced a DVD to inform young men about why and how they should carry out testicular self-examination, and publications describing scientific and clinical research findings. Orchid was involved in setting up the Experimental Cancer Medicine Centre at St Bart's and the Royal London School of Medicine.

Ovacome

www.ovacome.org.uk

Ovacome is a nationwide support network for everyone affected by ovarian cancer, including sufferers, friends, families, carers and health professionals. It aims to share experiences; link sufferers; provide information on treatments, screening and research; and raise awareness of the condition.

Patients Association

www.patients-association.com

Helpline: 0845 608 4455

The Patients Association aims to empower patients by listening to their concerns. It campaigns to improve services, provides access to advice and information, and works together with both patients and healthcare professionals.

Penny Brohn Cancer Care

www.pennybrohncancercare.org

Formerly the Bristol Cancer Help Centre, Penny Brohn Cancer Care offers specialist support including complementary therapies, advice and counselling for people living with cancer and their supporters. All services are offered free of charge.

Prostate Cancer Charity

www.prostate-cancer.org.uk

Helpline: 0800 074 8383

The charity fights prostate cancer through research, support, information and campaigning. It provides specialist information and support for men affected by prostate cancer and their families and friends.

Rare Cancer Alliance

www.rare-cancer.org

The Rare Cancer Alliance shares information and provides support to all paediatric (childhood) and rare cancer patients. Most of the members are patients or survivors, not medical professionals, and they hope their organisation and website will save patients some precious time and energy when trying to find out about their own rare cancers. They also raise awareness and funds for rare cancer research.

Rarer Cancers Foundation

www.rarercancers.org.uk

Helpline: 0800 434 6476

The Rarer Cancers Forum offers general advice and information and, where possible, patient-to-patient support. It collects up-to-date information, and puts patients with rare and less common cancers in contact with one another. It raises awareness about these cancers and tries to secure the best possible services for people living with rarer cancers.

Roy Castle Lung Cancer Foundation

www.roycastle.org

Helpline: 0800 358 7200

The Foundation is the only UK charity dedicated to defeating lung cancer. It funds lung cancer research, provides support, helps people to give up smoking and gives a voice to all those affected by the disease.

Tak Tent Cancer Support

www.cancersupportscotland.org

Tel: 0141 211 0122

'Tak Tent' comes from Old Scots and means 'take care'. The organisation was founded by Sir Kenneth Calman and aims to promote the care of cancer patients, their family and friends by providing emotional support to all. Tak Tent runs a network of support groups across Scotland, meeting monthly in the evening, including a group specifically for people aged 16–25. It also provides counselling and complementary therapies.

Tenovus Cancer Charity

www.tenovus.com

Helpline: 0808 808 1010

Tenovus is a charitable organisation based in Cardiff committed to the control of cancer through: quality research, prevention, education, counselling and patient care.

Ulster Cancer Foundation

www.ulstercancer.org

Helpline: 0800 783 3339

The Foundation aims to help all those who are affected by cancer. It provides an information, counselling and support unit; a telephone helpline; home and hospital visits; an information and referral service and support groups for specific cancers.

Urostomy Association

www.urostomyassociation.org.uk

Helpline: 08452 412159

The Association was formed to assist people who are about to undergo or have had surgery involving a urinary diversion. It offers wide-ranging counselling and advice, local meetings, hospital and home visits and twice-yearly journal. It also promotes and co-ordinates research.

Wessex Cancer Trust

www.wessexcancer.org

The Wessex Cancer Trust operates throughout Dorset, Hampshire, Wiltshire, the Isle of Wight and the Channel Islands. It promotes understanding and awareness of the disease and its effects by producing a wide range of leaflets. It also funds research, facilities for early detection and screening, and the promotion of cancer prevention. It has two seaside holiday homes for patients.

World Cancer Research Fund

www.wcrf-uk.org

Tel: 020 7343 4205

World Cancer Research Fund (WCRF UK) supports research into the role of diet and nutrition in the prevention of cancer. It also offers a wide range of cancer prevention education programmes and publications for health professionals, schools and the public. Through these pioneering efforts, WCRF UK has helped focus attention on the link between cancer and the choices made about food, drink, physical activity and bodyweight.

Index